# The Pancreatic Oath

## Nutrition & Lifestyle Journal

*Your Tool for an Effective Data-Driven Diet*

### Based on the Success of the
### Pancreatic Nutritional Program™

Candice P. Rosen, R.N., B.S., M.S.W., C.H.C.

For information about this title or to order other books and/or electronic media, contact the publisher:

Pancreatic Nutritional Program, a division of Candice Rosen Health Counseling, LLC

info@pnprogram.com

www.pnprogram.com <http://www.pnprogram.com>

Library of Congress Cataloguing-in-Publication Data

Rosen, Candice P.

Pancreatic Oath Nutrition & Lifestyle Journal, The: measurable approach to improved health and weight loss/Candice P. Rosen

ISBN: 978-0-9836413-2-2 Softcover

Printed in the United States of America

Cover and interior design: 1106 Design

*This book is dedicated to*

*Melissa,*
*Jennifer,*
*Natalie, and*
*Nicholas.*

*My reasons for being.*

# Table of Contents

# Your First Assignment

1. Go to the full-length mirror in your house.
2. Lock the doors to the room.
3. Take off all your clothes.
4. Examine your naked body in the mirror.

What do you see? What is your body trying to tell you?

Like a detective, comb your body visually for evidence of what conditions it is trying to alert you to. Look for outward manifestations of what is occurring internally.

Look at your stomach, your thighs, your butt, your face, upper arms, etc. What do they tell you?

Are there bulges in all the wrong places? Blatant obesity? Or even just a bloated appearance to your face? Double chin? Triple chin? Cystic acne? Wounds that are slow to heal or have left scars? Do you have skin tags or skin discoloration? Do you have to lift skin to wash? Do you have excessive unwanted hair or increased hair growth? Circles under your eyes?

This is not meant to induce shame—it is meant to begin a dialogue with your body. The mirror is one of the three voices your body has to speak to you. If your body looks "abused" in anyway, it is time for you to listen to it and help it. You can help stop the abuse by eating wisely and exercising. Your body is alerting you to the damage you are causing to your health through your current consumption habits. You must respond to its messages if you are going to get in shape and feel better.

*Please join me in protecting your pancreas,*
*a fundamental necessity for a future of*
*improved health and weight loss.*
*— Candice Rosen*

# Why Journal

1. Journaling is a way to maintain accountability. It keeps you honest.
2. The foundation of the Pancreatic Nutritional Program is discovering the connection between your diet, lifestyle, stress level and its impact on your blood glucose level.
3. You need to record data daily in order for the program to be effective and give you a clear picture of what foods and activities support pancreatic health as well as protect the pancreas, provide weight loss and improve health.
4. Take your journal everywhere or login to our online journal at www.ILOVEMYPANCREAS.COM to track your progress and ultimately, create the best nutrition and lifestyle management program for yourself.

In the beginning, you may feel like journaling is tedious or a waste of time. Change is rarely easy, but the first step is to commit to a meal-by-meal and day-by-day review of your diet and lifestyle. Your journal should be your place to confide and keep things "real." There is no point in lying about what you ate, how much you exercised or fibbing as to what your blood glucose numbers are in a given day. You will only be serving as a roadblock to your best self.

If you are honest in your journal and you commit to testing and recording your data daily, you will see patterns emerge as to what is pancreatic friendly and what is abusive to your pancreas. Tarot readers often describe psychic card readings as your soul's way of speaking to you. Well, what you record in your journal can be viewed as your body's way of communicating to you. It is a miraculous instrument that can and does survive much mistreatment on our parts.

However, if we want to honor our physical existences, we must learn from our bodies. What foods and beverages are positive for our particular body and what foods are negative. What our bodies prefer and do not prefer to consume. With a healthy diet, active lifestyle and investment in stress management and holistic personal care, we are giving our bodies the tools needed to heal and be well. We cannot just rely on our physician to rescue us by prescribing medications that mask symptoms, rather than addressing the root cause—the overconsumption of poor food choices coupled with a sedentary lifestyle. We must do our part to improve the state of our health and should look at ourselves as partners with our healthcare providers. We play a vital role in our own wellbeing. Please join me in practicing SELF-HEALTH.

> *Effective health care depends on self-care; this fact is currently heralded as if it were a discovery.*
> —*Ivan Illich*

## The Pancreatic Nutritional Program (PNP)™ Journal Instructions:

**Date:** Enter the date as well as the day of the week in this section. This will help you to determine patterns in your diet, activity and stress levels.

**Morning Blood Glucose:** Should be taken first thing in the morning after you wake up in a fasting state (before you have eaten or had anything to drink). Ideally, right after you use the bathroom and wash your hands, you should test your blood glucose.

**Weight:** Weigh yourself first thing in the morning after using the bathroom and before you have consumed any food or drink. Always weigh yourself completely naked and make sure the scale is in the same spot on a solid surface (no carpeting).

**Cup of Hot Water:** A mug of warmed water with a squeeze of lemon is beneficial for detoxification and stimulating the bowels.

**Meal Chart:** Record everything you ate and drank for each meal or snack. Record the time you ate. Approximately, 90 minutes later you will test your blood glucose to see the effects of what you ate and drank on your pancreas. To remind yourself when to test add 90 minutes to when you finished eating a meal or snack and place it in the "Time + 1.5 Hours Column." Note which meals and snacks keep your blood glucose within a healthy range.

*Speak and work with your physician. If you are a Type 1 or Type 2 Diabetic, your need for insulin or oral hypoglycemic agents will change as you improve your diet and lifestyle and lower your blood glucose. Diabetics should be vigilant about monitoring their lowering blood glucose levels. NEVER allow levels to go below 65.* Pancreas-friendly meals keep your blood glucose between: 70–100. Diabetics may range between 80–140. Remember—*the ultimate goal for diabetics are numbers closer to 100.*

**Stress Level:** High stress levels can have an adverse effect on blood glucose levels and your long-term health. It is important to monitor patterns of stress and develop management techniques. From the scale of 1–10 (with 10 being the most stressed), choose your overall stress level for the day.

**Exercise:** Moderate exercise is advocated on the PNP. Record your physical activity for the day. Monitor over time what variety of exercise works best for your body.

**Meditation/Deep Breathing:** Everyday you should take time to reflect and settle your mind, freeing it from family, work and other distractions. Aim for 10–20 minutes a day. In addition, deep cleansing breaths in the morning, at night or whenever needed are effective in managing stress and connecting you with gratitude for the miraculous functioning of your body.

**Vitamins:** Vitamins are beneficial support tools to your nutrition program. A list of *recommended* supplements may be found on page 88 in *The Pancreatic Oath: The Measurable Approach to Improved Health and Weight Loss.*

**Eight Glasses of Water:** Proper hydration is crucial to maintaining overall health and achieving weight loss.

# The Pancreatic Oath

*I promise to cherish, protect, respect, and nourish my pancreas and my body.*

*I will abstain from food, drink, and substances that place a burden or have a destructive effect on my pancreas, my body, my mind and my spirit.*

*I will take responsibility and do all in my power to improve and maintain my health and to prevent illness. I make this pledge not only for me, but also for those entrusted with my care.*

## Oaths to My Body, Mind and Spirit

Please list pledges you are willing to make to improve your health and wellbeing.

1. _____

   _____

2. _____

   _____

3. _____

   _____

4. _____

   _____

5. _____

   _____

6. _____

   _____

7. _____

   _____

8. _____

   _____

9. _____

   _____

10. _____

    _____

## The Ten Commandments of Good Health

1. Thou shall protect the pancreas.
2. Thou shall avoid processed foods.
3. Thou shall maintain a healthy glucose level.
4. Thou shall exercise and meditate.
5. Thou shall practice proper food combinations.
6. Thou shall read food labels.
7. Thou shall practice portion control.
8. Thou shall eliminate sugars.
9. Thou shall eat fruit separately.
10. Thou shall love, cherish and protect thy health.

# Results

BEFORE PICTURE

AFTER PICTURE

DATE: _____

DATE (12 WEEKS AFTER
THE START DATE): _____

*He who has health, has hope.*
*And he who has hope, has everything.*
*—Arab Proverb*

# PNP Health Transformation Progress Report

*The greatest of follies is to sacrifice health
for any other kind of happiness.*
*—Arthur Schopenhauer*

**BEFORE Measurements:**

Weight _____

Chest _____

Left Upper Arm _____

Right Upper Arm _____

Waist _____

Hips _____

Left Upper Thigh _____

Right Upper Thigh _____

Left Ankle _____

Right Ankle _____

**AFTER Measurements:**
(12 Weeks After Start Date)

Weight _____

Chest _____

Left Upper Arm _____

Right Upper Arm _____

Waist _____

Hips _____

Left Upper Thigh _____

Right Upper Thigh _____

Left Ankle _____

Right Ankle _____

*Give a man health and a course to steer,
and he'll never stop to trouble about
whether he's happy or not.*
*—George Bernard Shaw*

# Pancreatic Nutritional Program (PNP)™ Fasting Blood Work Review

> *The awareness that health is dependent upon habits that we control makes us the first generation in history that to a large extent determines its own destiny.*
> *—Jimmy Carter*

**BEFORE:**

**Fasting Blood Glucose** _____

**Lipid panel** _____

- Total Cholesterol _____

- HDL Cholesterol _____

- LDL Cholesterol _____

- Triglycerides _____

**Comprehensive metabolic panel (CMP)** _____

- Chloride _____

- Sodium _____

- $CO_2$ _____

- Potassium _____

- Calcium _____

- Glucose _____

- BUN _____

- Creatinine _____
- Total Protein _____
- Total Bilirubin _____
- Albumin _____
- Alkaline Phosphatase _____
- Aspartate Aminotransferase _____
- Alanine Aminotransferase _____

**Thyroid function** _____

- T3 _____
- Total T4 _____
- Free T4 _____
- Thyroid Stimulating Hormone (TSH) _____

**Complete blood count (CBC)** _____

- White blood cell count (WBC or leukocyte count) _____
- WBC differential count _____
- Red blood cell count (RBC or erythrocyte count) _____
- Hematocrit (Hct) _____
- Hemoglobin (Hbg) _____
- Mean corpuscular volume (MCV) _____
- Mean corpuscular hemoglobin (MCH) _____
- Mean corpuscular hemoglobin concentration (MCHC) _____
- Red cell distribution width (RDW) _____

- Platelet count _____

- Mean Platelet Volume (MPV) _____

**Women** _____
(Specifically Adolescent and Adult females suspected of suffering from symptoms of polycystic ovarian syndrome—PCOS)

- Follicle Stimulating Hormone (FSH) _____

- Luteinizing Hormone (LH) _____

- Testosterone levels _____

**Men** _____
(Especially for men suffering from erectile dysfunction)

- Testosterone levels _____

> *A man's health can be judged by which he takes*
> *two at a time—pills or stairs.*
> *—Joan Welsh*

**AFTER (12 Weeks After Start Date):**

**Fasting Blood Glucose** _____

**Lipid panel** _____

- Total Cholesterol _____

- HDL Cholesterol _____

- LDL Cholesterol _____

- Triglycerides _____

**Comprehensive metabolic panel (CMP)** _____

- Chloride _____

- Sodium _____

- $CO_2$ _____

- Potassium _____

- Calcium _____

- Glucose _____

- BUN _____

- Creatinine _____

- Total Protein _____

- Total Bilirubin _____

- Albumin _____

- Alkaline Phosphatase _____

- Aspartate Aminotransferase _____

- Alanine Aminotransferase _____

**Thyroid function** _____

- T3 _____

- Total T4 _____

- Free T4 _____

- Thyroid Stimulating Hormone (TSH) _____

**Complete blood count (CBC)** _____

- White blood cell count (WBC or leukocyte count) _____

- WBC differential count _____
- Red blood cell count (RBC or erythrocyte count) _____
- Hematocrit (Hct) _____
- Hemoglobin (Hbg) _____
- Mean corpuscular volume (MCV) _____
- Mean corpuscular hemoglobin (MCH) _____
- Mean corpuscular hemoglobin concentration (MCHC) _____
- Red cell distribution width (RDW) _____
- Platelet count _____
- Mean Platelet Volume (MPV) _____

**Women** _____
(Specifically Adolescent and Adult females suspected of suffering from symptoms of polycystic ovarian syndrome—PCOS)

- Follicle Stimulating Hormone (FSH) _____
- Luteinizing Hormone (LH) _____
- Testosterone levels _____

**Men** _____
(Especially for men suffering from erectile dysfunction)

- Testosterone levels _____

*Good health and good sense are two*
*of life's greatest blessings.*
*—Publilius Syrus*

## Goal Blood Glucose Ranges

*A wise man should consider that health is the greatest of human blessings, and learn how by his own thought to derive benefit from his illnesses.*
*—Hippocrates*

**Non-Diabetics:** 70–100

**Diabetics:** 80–140

*Speak and work with your physician. It is an important partnership. ATTENTION DIABETICS: Your need for insulin or oral hypoglycemic agents will change as you improve your diet, activity and lifestyle choices. You should be vigilant about both monitoring and lowering glucose levels. NEVER allow levels to go below 65. The ultimate goal for diabetics are numbers closer to 100.*

## Portion Sizes

Piece or cup of Fruit—Baseball
3 oz. portion of tofu, tempeh, fish, chicken, eggs or meat—Deck of Cards
½ cup of lentils, beans, pasta or rice—Baseball
1 tablespoon of nut butter—1 large thumb tip
One serving of nuts—10 to 12 nuts

*The preservation of health is a duty. Few seem conscious that there is such a thing as physical morality.*
*—Herbert Spencer*

# Journal Pages

A man too busy to take care of his health is like a
mechanic too busy to take care of his tools.
—*Spanish Proverb*

In health there is freedom.
Health is the first of all liberties.
—*Henri Frederic Amiel*

## LIFE GOALS . . . for the First 4 Weeks

The simple task of listing your goals has a powerful effect on organizing your priorities and helping you to achieve your health, career and happiness desires.

1. List goals in the numbered spaces.
2. Under each goal—list three action steps necessary on YOUR part to achieve the written goal.
3. Once an action step or a goal is achieved, cross it off with a red pen.

GOAL 1: _____

    Action Step A: _____

    Action Step B: _____

    Action Step C: _____

GOAL 2: _____

    Action Step A: _____

    Action Step B: _____

    Action Step C: _____

GOAL 3: _____

    Action Step A: _____

    Action Step B: _____

    Action Step C: _____

GOAL 4: _____

    Action Step A: _____

    Action Step B: _____

    Action Step C: _____

GOAL 5: _____

    Action Step A: _____

    Action Step B: _____

    Action Step C: _____

GOAL 6: _____

    Action Step A: _____

    Action Step B: _____

    Action Step C: _____

GOAL 7: _____

    Action Step A: _____

    Action Step B: _____

    Action Step C: _____

DATE _____

MORNING BLOOD GLUCOSE _____

WEIGHT _____

CUP OF HOT WATER          Yes     No

|  | Meal | Time | Time + 1.5 hours | Glucose at 1.5 hours |
|---|---|---|---|---|
| Breakfast |  |  |  |  |
| Snack |  |  |  |  |
| Lunch |  |  |  |  |
| Snack |  |  |  |  |
| Dinner |  |  |  |  |

STRESS LEVEL _____

Low ⟶ High

1     2     3     4     5     6     7     8     9     10

EXERCISE   Type _____          Yes     No

MEDITATION/DEEP BREATHING                       Yes     No

VITAMIN                                          Yes     No

EIGHT GLASSES OF WATER                           Yes     No

DATE _____

MORNING BLOOD GLUCOSE _____

WEIGHT _____

CUP OF HOT WATER          Yes     No

| | Meal | Time | Time + 1.5 hours | Glucose at 1.5 hours |
|---|---|---|---|---|
| Breakfast | | | | |
| Snack | | | | |
| Lunch | | | | |
| Snack | | | | |
| Dinner | | | | |

STRESS LEVEL _____

Low ————————————————————————▶ High

    1     2     3     4     5     6     7     8     9    10

EXERCISE  Type _____          Yes     No

MEDITATION/DEEP BREATHING                         Yes     No

VITAMIN                                           Yes     No

EIGHT GLASSES OF WATER                            Yes     No

DATE _____

MORNING BLOOD GLUCOSE _____

WEIGHT _____

CUP OF HOT WATER          Yes     No

|  | Meal | Time | Time + 1.5 hours | Glucose at 1.5 hours |
|---|---|---|---|---|
| Breakfast |  |  |  |  |
| Snack |  |  |  |  |
| Lunch |  |  |  |  |
| Snack |  |  |  |  |
| Dinner |  |  |  |  |

STRESS LEVEL _____

Low  ————————————————————➤  High

1     2     3     4     5     6     7     8     9     10

EXERCISE   Type _____          Yes     No

MEDITATION/DEEP BREATHING          Yes     No

VITAMIN          Yes     No

EIGHT GLASSES OF WATER          Yes     No

DATE _____

MORNING BLOOD GLUCOSE _____

WEIGHT _____

CUP OF HOT WATER        Yes    No

| | Meal | Time | Time + 1.5 hours | Glucose at 1.5 hours |
|---|---|---|---|---|
| Breakfast | | | | |
| Snack | | | | |
| Lunch | | | | |
| Snack | | | | |
| Dinner | | | | |

STRESS LEVEL _____

Low ──────────────────────→ High

1    2    3    4    5    6    7    8    9    10

EXERCISE  Type _____        Yes    No

MEDITATION/DEEP BREATHING                     Yes    No

VITAMIN                                        Yes    No

EIGHT GLASSES OF WATER                         Yes    No

DATE _____

MORNING BLOOD GLUCOSE _____

WEIGHT _____

CUP OF HOT WATER          Yes     No

|  | Meal | Time | Time + 1.5 hours | Glucose at 1.5 hours |
|---|---|---|---|---|
| Breakfast |  |  |  |  |
| Snack |  |  |  |  |
| Lunch |  |  |  |  |
| Snack |  |  |  |  |
| Dinner |  |  |  |  |

STRESS LEVEL _____

Low ——————————————————→ High

  1    2    3    4    5    6    7    8    9    10

EXERCISE   Type _____          Yes     No

MEDITATION/DEEP BREATHING                             Yes     No

VITAMIN                                                              Yes     No

EIGHT GLASSES OF WATER                                  Yes     No

DATE _____

MORNING BLOOD GLUCOSE _____

WEIGHT _____

CUP OF HOT WATER          Yes    No

| | Meal | Time | Time + 1.5 hours | Glucose at 1.5 hours |
|---|---|---|---|---|
| Breakfast | | | | |
| Snack | | | | |
| Lunch | | | | |
| Snack | | | | |
| Dinner | | | | |

STRESS LEVEL _____

Low ————————————————————▶ High

1    2    3    4    5    6    7    8    9    10

EXERCISE  Type _____          Yes     No

MEDITATION/DEEP BREATHING                        Yes     No

VITAMIN                                          Yes     No

EIGHT GLASSES OF WATER                           Yes     No

DATE _____

MORNING BLOOD GLUCOSE _____

WEIGHT _____

CUP OF HOT WATER          Yes     No

| | Meal | Time | Time + 1.5 hours | Glucose at 1.5 hours |
|---|---|---|---|---|
| Breakfast | | | | |
| Snack | | | | |
| Lunch | | | | |
| Snack | | | | |
| Dinner | | | | |

STRESS LEVEL _____

Low ⟶ High

1     2     3     4     5     6     7     8     9     10

EXERCISE   Type _____          Yes     No

MEDITATION/DEEP BREATHING                              Yes     No

VITAMIN                                                Yes     No

EIGHT GLASSES OF WATER                                 Yes     No

DATE _____

MORNING BLOOD GLUCOSE _____

WEIGHT _____

CUP OF HOT WATER          Yes     No

|  | Meal | Time | Time +<br>1.5 hours | Glucose at<br>1.5 hours |
|---|---|---|---|---|
| Breakfast |  |  |  |  |
| Snack |  |  |  |  |
| Lunch |  |  |  |  |
| Snack |  |  |  |  |
| Dinner |  |  |  |  |

STRESS LEVEL _____

Low  ————————————————————————▶  High

   1      2      3      4      5      6      7      8      9     10

EXERCISE  Type _____          Yes     No

MEDITATION/DEEP BREATHING                          Yes     No

VITAMIN                                            Yes     No

EIGHT GLASSES OF WATER                             Yes     No

DATE _____

MORNING BLOOD GLUCOSE _____

WEIGHT _____

CUP OF HOT WATER          Yes    No

|  | Meal | Time | Time + 1.5 hours | Glucose at 1.5 hours |
|---|---|---|---|---|
| Breakfast |  |  |  |  |
| Snack |  |  |  |  |
| Lunch |  |  |  |  |
| Snack |  |  |  |  |
| Dinner |  |  |  |  |

STRESS LEVEL _____

Low ⟶ High

1     2     3     4     5     6     7     8     9     10

EXERCISE   Type _____          Yes    No

MEDITATION/DEEP BREATHING                       Yes    No

VITAMIN                                          Yes    No

EIGHT GLASSES OF WATER                           Yes    No

DATE _____

MORNING BLOOD GLUCOSE _____

WEIGHT _____

CUP OF HOT WATER          Yes     No

|  | Meal | Time | Time + 1.5 hours | Glucose at 1.5 hours |
|---|---|---|---|---|
| Breakfast |  |  |  |  |
| Snack |  |  |  |  |
| Lunch |  |  |  |  |
| Snack |  |  |  |  |
| Dinner |  |  |  |  |

STRESS LEVEL _____

Low ──────────────────────────▶ High
1      2      3      4      5      6      7      8      9      10

EXERCISE   Type _____          Yes     No

MEDITATION/DEEP BREATHING          Yes     No

VITAMIN          Yes     No

EIGHT GLASSES OF WATER          Yes     No

DATE _____

MORNING BLOOD GLUCOSE _____

WEIGHT _____

CUP OF HOT WATER          Yes     No

|  | Meal | Time | Time + 1.5 hours | Glucose at 1.5 hours |
|---|---|---|---|---|
| Breakfast |  |  |  |  |
| Snack |  |  |  |  |
| Lunch |  |  |  |  |
| Snack |  |  |  |  |
| Dinner |  |  |  |  |

STRESS LEVEL _____

Low  ———————————————————➤  High

  1    2    3    4    5    6    7    8    9    10

EXERCISE   Type _____          Yes     No

MEDITATION/DEEP BREATHING                              Yes     No

VITAMIN                                                Yes     No

EIGHT GLASSES OF WATER                                 Yes     No

DATE _____

MORNING BLOOD GLUCOSE _____

WEIGHT _____

CUP OF HOT WATER          Yes     No

|  | Meal | Time | Time + 1.5 hours | Glucose at 1.5 hours |
|---|---|---|---|---|
| Breakfast |  |  |  |  |
| Snack |  |  |  |  |
| Lunch |  |  |  |  |
| Snack |  |  |  |  |
| Dinner |  |  |  |  |

STRESS LEVEL _____

Low  ————————————————————→  High
  1    2    3    4    5    6    7    8    9    10

EXERCISE  Type _____          Yes     No

MEDITATION/DEEP BREATHING                        Yes     No

VITAMIN                                          Yes     No

EIGHT GLASSES OF WATER                           Yes     No

DATE _____

MORNING BLOOD GLUCOSE _____

WEIGHT _____

CUP OF HOT WATER          Yes    No

|  | Meal | Time | Time + 1.5 hours | Glucose at 1.5 hours |
|---|---|---|---|---|
| Breakfast |  |  |  |  |
| Snack |  |  |  |  |
| Lunch |  |  |  |  |
| Snack |  |  |  |  |
| Dinner |  |  |  |  |

STRESS LEVEL _____

Low ⟶ High

1     2     3     4     5     6     7     8     9     10

EXERCISE   Type _____          Yes     No

MEDITATION/DEEP BREATHING                          Yes     No

VITAMIN                                             Yes     No

EIGHT GLASSES OF WATER                             Yes     No

DATE _____

MORNING BLOOD GLUCOSE _____

WEIGHT _____

CUP OF HOT WATER     Yes    No

|  | Meal | Time | Time + 1.5 hours | Glucose at 1.5 hours |
|---|---|---|---|---|
| Breakfast |  |  |  |  |
| Snack |  |  |  |  |
| Lunch |  |  |  |  |
| Snack |  |  |  |  |
| Dinner |  |  |  |  |

STRESS LEVEL _____

Low ⟶ High

1    2    3    4    5    6    7    8    9    10

EXERCISE  Type _____     Yes    No

MEDITATION/DEEP BREATHING                Yes    No

VITAMIN                                  Yes    No

EIGHT GLASSES OF WATER                   Yes    No

DATE _____

MORNING BLOOD GLUCOSE _____

WEIGHT _____

CUP OF HOT WATER          Yes    No

|  | Meal | Time | Time + 1.5 hours | Glucose at 1.5 hours |
|---|---|---|---|---|
| Breakfast |  |  |  |  |
| Snack |  |  |  |  |
| Lunch |  |  |  |  |
| Snack |  |  |  |  |
| Dinner |  |  |  |  |

STRESS LEVEL _____

Low ⟶ High

  1      2      3      4      5      6      7      8      9     10

EXERCISE  Type _____          Yes      No

MEDITATION/DEEP BREATHING                        Yes      No

VITAMIN                                          Yes      No

EIGHT GLASSES OF WATER                           Yes      No

DATE _____

MORNING BLOOD GLUCOSE _____

WEIGHT _____

CUP OF HOT WATER          Yes    No

|  | Meal | Time | Time + 1.5 hours | Glucose at 1.5 hours |
|---|---|---|---|---|
| Breakfast |  |  |  |  |
| Snack |  |  |  |  |
| Lunch |  |  |  |  |
| Snack |  |  |  |  |
| Dinner |  |  |  |  |

STRESS LEVEL _____

Low  ————————————————————▶  High

1    2    3    4    5    6    7    8    9    10

EXERCISE   Type _____          Yes    No

MEDITATION/DEEP BREATHING          Yes    No

VITAMIN          Yes    No

EIGHT GLASSES OF WATER          Yes    No

DATE _____

MORNING BLOOD GLUCOSE _____

WEIGHT _____

CUP OF HOT WATER          Yes     No

|  | Meal | Time | Time + 1.5 hours | Glucose at 1.5 hours |
|---|---|---|---|---|
| Breakfast |  |  |  |  |
| Snack |  |  |  |  |
| Lunch |  |  |  |  |
| Snack |  |  |  |  |
| Dinner |  |  |  |  |

STRESS LEVEL _____

Low ⎯⎯⎯⎯⎯⎯⎯⎯⎯⎯⎯⎯⎯⎯⎯⎯→ High

  1     2     3     4     5     6     7     8     9     10

EXERCISE   Type _____          Yes     No

MEDITATION/DEEP BREATHING                         Yes     No

VITAMIN                                           Yes     No

EIGHT GLASSES OF WATER                            Yes     No

DATE _____

MORNING BLOOD GLUCOSE _____

WEIGHT _____

CUP OF HOT WATER          Yes    No

|  | Meal | Time | Time + 1.5 hours | Glucose at 1.5 hours |
|---|---|---|---|---|
| Breakfast |  |  |  |  |
| Snack |  |  |  |  |
| Lunch |  |  |  |  |
| Snack |  |  |  |  |
| Dinner |  |  |  |  |

STRESS LEVEL _____

Low ⟶ High

1    2    3    4    5    6    7    8    9    10

EXERCISE   Type _____          Yes    No

MEDITATION/DEEP BREATHING               Yes    No

VITAMIN                                  Yes    No

EIGHT GLASSES OF WATER                   Yes    No

DATE  _____

MORNING BLOOD GLUCOSE  _____

WEIGHT  _____

CUP OF HOT WATER          Yes     No

| | Meal | Time | Time + 1.5 hours | Glucose at 1.5 hours |
|---|---|---|---|---|
| Breakfast | | | | |
| Snack | | | | |
| Lunch | | | | |
| Snack | | | | |
| Dinner | | | | |

STRESS LEVEL  _____

Low  ————————————————————➤  High

  1    2    3    4    5    6    7    8    9   10

EXERCISE   Type _____          Yes     No

MEDITATION/DEEP BREATHING          Yes     No

VITAMIN          Yes     No

EIGHT GLASSES OF WATER          Yes     No

DATE _____

MORNING BLOOD GLUCOSE _____

WEIGHT _____

CUP OF HOT WATER       Yes   No

| | Meal | Time | Time + 1.5 hours | Glucose at 1.5 hours |
|---|---|---|---|---|
| Breakfast | | | | |
| Snack | | | | |
| Lunch | | | | |
| Snack | | | | |
| Dinner | | | | |

STRESS LEVEL _____

Low  ————————————————————▶  High

  1    2    3    4    5    6    7    8    9   10

EXERCISE  Type _____     Yes   No

MEDITATION/DEEP BREATHING     Yes   No

VITAMIN     Yes   No

EIGHT GLASSES OF WATER     Yes   No

DATE _____

MORNING BLOOD GLUCOSE _____

WEIGHT _____

CUP OF HOT WATER          Yes     No

|  | Meal | Time | Time + 1.5 hours | Glucose at 1.5 hours |
|---|---|---|---|---|
| Breakfast |  |  |  |  |
| Snack |  |  |  |  |
| Lunch |  |  |  |  |
| Snack |  |  |  |  |
| Dinner |  |  |  |  |

STRESS LEVEL _____

Low ————————————————————→ High

1     2     3     4     5     6     7     8     9     10

EXERCISE   Type _____          Yes     No

MEDITATION/DEEP BREATHING                          Yes     No

VITAMIN                                            Yes     No

EIGHT GLASSES OF WATER                             Yes     No

DATE _____

MORNING BLOOD GLUCOSE _____

WEIGHT _____

CUP OF HOT WATER          Yes     No

|  | Meal | Time | Time + 1.5 hours | Glucose at 1.5 hours |
|---|---|---|---|---|
| Breakfast |  |  |  |  |
| Snack |  |  |  |  |
| Lunch |  |  |  |  |
| Snack |  |  |  |  |
| Dinner |  |  |  |  |

STRESS LEVEL _____

Low ⟶ High

| 1 | 2 | 3 | 4 | 5 | 6 | 7 | 8 | 9 | 10 |

EXERCISE  Type _____          Yes     No

MEDITATION/DEEP BREATHING                Yes     No

VITAMIN                                  Yes     No

EIGHT GLASSES OF WATER                   Yes     No

DATE _____

MORNING BLOOD GLUCOSE _____

WEIGHT _____

CUP OF HOT WATER          Yes    No

|  | Meal | Time | Time + 1.5 hours | Glucose at 1.5 hours |
|---|---|---|---|---|
| Breakfast |  |  |  |  |
| Snack |  |  |  |  |
| Lunch |  |  |  |  |
| Snack |  |  |  |  |
| Dinner |  |  |  |  |

STRESS LEVEL _____

Low ———————————————————➤ High

1    2    3    4    5    6    7    8    9    10

EXERCISE  Type _____          Yes    No

MEDITATION/DEEP BREATHING                    Yes    No

VITAMIN                                       Yes    No

EIGHT GLASSES OF WATER                        Yes    No

DATE _____

MORNING BLOOD GLUCOSE _____

WEIGHT _____

CUP OF HOT WATER          Yes      No

|  | Meal | Time | Time + 1.5 hours | Glucose at 1.5 hours |
|---|---|---|---|---|
| Breakfast |  |  |  |  |
| Snack |  |  |  |  |
| Lunch |  |  |  |  |
| Snack |  |  |  |  |
| Dinner |  |  |  |  |

STRESS LEVEL _____

Low ————————————————————➔ High

1      2      3      4      5      6      7      8      9      10

EXERCISE   Type _____          Yes      No

MEDITATION/DEEP BREATHING          Yes      No

VITAMIN          Yes      No

EIGHT GLASSES OF WATER          Yes      No

DATE _____

MORNING BLOOD GLUCOSE _____

WEIGHT _____

CUP OF HOT WATER          Yes     No

|  | Meal | Time | Time + 1.5 hours | Glucose at 1.5 hours |
|---|---|---|---|---|
| Breakfast |  |  |  |  |
| Snack |  |  |  |  |
| Lunch |  |  |  |  |
| Snack |  |  |  |  |
| Dinner |  |  |  |  |

STRESS LEVEL _____

Low ————————————————→ High

1     2     3     4     5     6     7     8     9     10

| EXERCISE  Type _____ | Yes | No |
|---|---|---|
| MEDITATION/DEEP BREATHING | Yes | No |
| VITAMIN | Yes | No |
| EIGHT GLASSES OF WATER | Yes | No |

DATE _____

MORNING BLOOD GLUCOSE _____

WEIGHT _____

CUP OF HOT WATER          Yes    No

|  | Meal | Time | Time + 1.5 hours | Glucose at 1.5 hours |
|---|---|---|---|---|
| Breakfast |  |  |  |  |
| Snack |  |  |  |  |
| Lunch |  |  |  |  |
| Snack |  |  |  |  |
| Dinner |  |  |  |  |

STRESS LEVEL _____

Low ——————————————————→ High

1    2    3    4    5    6    7    8    9    10

EXERCISE   Type _____          Yes    No

MEDITATION/DEEP BREATHING                         Yes    No

VITAMIN                                           Yes    No

EIGHT GLASSES OF WATER                            Yes    No

DATE _____

MORNING BLOOD GLUCOSE _____

WEIGHT _____

CUP OF HOT WATER          Yes     No

|  | Meal | Time | Time + 1.5 hours | Glucose at 1.5 hours |
|---|---|---|---|---|
| Breakfast |  |  |  |  |
| Snack |  |  |  |  |
| Lunch |  |  |  |  |
| Snack |  |  |  |  |
| Dinner |  |  |  |  |

STRESS LEVEL _____

Low ——————————————————————➤ High
  1    2    3    4    5    6    7    8    9   10

EXERCISE   Type _____          Yes     No

MEDITATION/DEEP BREATHING          Yes     No

VITAMIN          Yes     No

EIGHT GLASSES OF WATER          Yes     No

DATE _____

MORNING BLOOD GLUCOSE _____

WEIGHT _____

CUP OF HOT WATER        Yes    No

| | Meal | Time | Time + 1.5 hours | Glucose at 1.5 hours |
|---|---|---|---|---|
| Breakfast | | | | |
| Snack | | | | |
| Lunch | | | | |
| Snack | | | | |
| Dinner | | | | |

STRESS LEVEL _____

Low ——————————————————→ High

1    2    3    4    5    6    7    8    9    10

EXERCISE  Type _____        Yes    No

MEDITATION/DEEP BREATHING        Yes    No

VITAMIN        Yes    No

EIGHT GLASSES OF WATER        Yes    No

## LIFE GOALS . . . for the Second 4 Weeks

The simple task of listing your goals has a powerful effect on organizing your priorities and helping you to achieve your health, career and happiness desires.

1.  List goals in the numbered spaces.
2.  Under each goal—list three action steps necessary on YOUR part to achieve the written goal.
3.  Once an action step or a goal is achieved, cross it off with a red pen.

GOAL 1: _____

    Action Step A: _____

    Action Step B: _____

    Action Step C: _____

GOAL 2: _____

    Action Step A: _____

    Action Step B: _____

    Action Step C: _____

GOAL 3: _____

    Action Step A: _____

    Action Step B: _____

    Action Step C: _____

GOAL 4: _____

    Action Step A: _____

    Action Step B: _____

    Action Step C: _____

GOAL 5: _____

    Action Step A: _____

    Action Step B: _____

    Action Step C: _____

GOAL 6: _____

    Action Step A: _____

    Action Step B: _____

    Action Step C: _____

GOAL 7: _____

    Action Step A: _____

    Action Step B: _____

    Action Step C: _____

DATE _____

MORNING BLOOD GLUCOSE _____

WEIGHT _____

CUP OF HOT WATER        Yes    No

|  | Meal | Time | Time + 1.5 hours | Glucose at 1.5 hours |
|---|---|---|---|---|
| Breakfast |  |  |  |  |
| Snack |  |  |  |  |
| Lunch |  |  |  |  |
| Snack |  |  |  |  |
| Dinner |  |  |  |  |

STRESS LEVEL _____

Low ——————————————————————→ High

  1     2     3     4     5     6     7     8     9    10

EXERCISE   Type _____        Yes    No

MEDITATION/DEEP BREATHING                       Yes    No

VITAMIN                                          Yes    No

EIGHT GLASSES OF WATER                           Yes    No

DATE _____

MORNING BLOOD GLUCOSE _____

WEIGHT _____

CUP OF HOT WATER          Yes     No

|  | Meal | Time | Time + 1.5 hours | Glucose at 1.5 hours |
|---|---|---|---|---|
| Breakfast |  |  |  |  |
| Snack |  |  |  |  |
| Lunch |  |  |  |  |
| Snack |  |  |  |  |
| Dinner |  |  |  |  |

STRESS LEVEL _____

Low ————————————————→ High

1     2     3     4     5     6     7     8     9     10

EXERCISE   Type _____          Yes     No

MEDITATION/DEEP BREATHING                         Yes     No

VITAMIN                                           Yes     No

EIGHT GLASSES OF WATER                            Yes     No

DATE _____

MORNING BLOOD GLUCOSE _____

WEIGHT _____

CUP OF HOT WATER          Yes     No

|  | Meal | Time | Time + 1.5 hours | Glucose at 1.5 hours |
|---|---|---|---|---|
| Breakfast |  |  |  |  |
| Snack |  |  |  |  |
| Lunch |  |  |  |  |
| Snack |  |  |  |  |
| Dinner |  |  |  |  |

STRESS LEVEL _____

Low ⟶ High

1    2    3    4    5    6    7    8    9    10

EXERCISE   Type _____          Yes     No

MEDITATION/DEEP BREATHING                              Yes     No

VITAMIN                                                Yes     No

EIGHT GLASSES OF WATER                                 Yes     No

DATE _____

MORNING BLOOD GLUCOSE _____

WEIGHT _____

CUP OF HOT WATER       Yes    No

|  | Meal | Time | Time + 1.5 hours | Glucose at 1.5 hours |
|---|---|---|---|---|
| Breakfast |  |  |  |  |
| Snack |  |  |  |  |
| Lunch |  |  |  |  |
| Snack |  |  |  |  |
| Dinner |  |  |  |  |

STRESS LEVEL _____

Low  ———————————————————————→  High

1     2     3     4     5     6     7     8     9     10

EXERCISE  Type _____           Yes    No

MEDITATION/DEEP BREATHING                       Yes    No

VITAMIN                                          Yes    No

EIGHT GLASSES OF WATER                           Yes    No

DATE _____

MORNING BLOOD GLUCOSE _____

WEIGHT _____

CUP OF HOT WATER          Yes     No

| | Meal | Time | Time + 1.5 hours | Glucose at 1.5 hours |
|---|---|---|---|---|
| Breakfast | | | | |
| Snack | | | | |
| Lunch | | | | |
| Snack | | | | |
| Dinner | | | | |

STRESS LEVEL _____

Low ————————————————————→ High
  1      2      3      4      5      6      7      8      9      10

EXERCISE   Type _____          Yes     No

MEDITATION/DEEP BREATHING                          Yes     No

VITAMIN                                            Yes     No

EIGHT GLASSES OF WATER                             Yes     No

DATE _____

MORNING BLOOD GLUCOSE _____

WEIGHT _____

CUP OF HOT WATER          Yes    No

|  | Meal | Time | Time + 1.5 hours | Glucose at 1.5 hours |
|---|---|---|---|---|
| Breakfast |  |  |  |  |
| Snack |  |  |  |  |
| Lunch |  |  |  |  |
| Snack |  |  |  |  |
| Dinner |  |  |  |  |

STRESS LEVEL _____

Low ————————————————————→ High

1     2     3     4     5     6     7     8     9     10

EXERCISE   Type _____          Yes    No

MEDITATION/DEEP BREATHING                         Yes    No

VITAMIN                                           Yes    No

EIGHT GLASSES OF WATER                            Yes    No

DATE _____

MORNING BLOOD GLUCOSE _____

WEIGHT _____

CUP OF HOT WATER          Yes     No

|  | Meal | Time | Time + 1.5 hours | Glucose at 1.5 hours |
|---|---|---|---|---|
| Breakfast |  |  |  |  |
| Snack |  |  |  |  |
| Lunch |  |  |  |  |
| Snack |  |  |  |  |
| Dinner |  |  |  |  |

STRESS LEVEL _____

Low ──────────────────────➤ High

   1     2     3     4     5     6     7     8     9     10

EXERCISE  Type _____          Yes     No

MEDITATION/DEEP BREATHING                         Yes     No

VITAMIN                                           Yes     No

EIGHT GLASSES OF WATER                            Yes     No

DATE _____

MORNING BLOOD GLUCOSE _____

WEIGHT _____

CUP OF HOT WATER          Yes    No

|  | Meal | Time | Time + 1.5 hours | Glucose at 1.5 hours |
|---|---|---|---|---|
| Breakfast |  |  |  |  |
| Snack |  |  |  |  |
| Lunch |  |  |  |  |
| Snack |  |  |  |  |
| Dinner |  |  |  |  |

STRESS LEVEL _____

Low ————————————————————→ High

1    2    3    4    5    6    7    8    9    10

EXERCISE  Type _____        Yes    No

MEDITATION/DEEP BREATHING                    Yes    No

VITAMIN                                      Yes    No

EIGHT GLASSES OF WATER                       Yes    No

DATE _____

MORNING BLOOD GLUCOSE _____

WEIGHT _____

CUP OF HOT WATER          Yes    No

|  | Meal | Time | Time + 1.5 hours | Glucose at 1.5 hours |
|---|---|---|---|---|
| Breakfast |  |  |  |  |
| Snack |  |  |  |  |
| Lunch |  |  |  |  |
| Snack |  |  |  |  |
| Dinner |  |  |  |  |

STRESS LEVEL _____

Low ————————————————➤ High

1    2    3    4    5    6    7    8    9    10

EXERCISE   Type _____          Yes    No

MEDITATION/DEEP BREATHING          Yes    No

VITAMIN          Yes    No

EIGHT GLASSES OF WATER          Yes    No

DATE _____

MORNING BLOOD GLUCOSE _____

WEIGHT _____

CUP OF HOT WATER          Yes    No

| | Meal | Time | Time + 1.5 hours | Glucose at 1.5 hours |
|---|---|---|---|---|
| Breakfast | | | | |
| Snack | | | | |
| Lunch | | | | |
| Snack | | | | |
| Dinner | | | | |

STRESS LEVEL _____

Low ——————————————————————► High

1      2      3      4      5      6      7      8      9      10

EXERCISE   Type _____          Yes    No

MEDITATION/DEEP BREATHING          Yes    No

VITAMIN          Yes    No

EIGHT GLASSES OF WATER          Yes    No

DATE _____

MORNING BLOOD GLUCOSE _____

WEIGHT _____

CUP OF HOT WATER          Yes     No

|  | Meal | Time | Time + 1.5 hours | Glucose at 1.5 hours |
|---|---|---|---|---|
| Breakfast |  |  |  |  |
| Snack |  |  |  |  |
| Lunch |  |  |  |  |
| Snack |  |  |  |  |
| Dinner |  |  |  |  |

STRESS LEVEL _____

Low  ⟶  High

1     2     3     4     5     6     7     8     9     10

| EXERCISE   Type _____ | Yes | No |
|---|---|---|
| MEDITATION/DEEP BREATHING | Yes | No |
| VITAMIN | Yes | No |
| EIGHT GLASSES OF WATER | Yes | No |

DATE _____

MORNING BLOOD GLUCOSE _____

WEIGHT _____

CUP OF HOT WATER          Yes     No

|  | Meal | Time | Time + 1.5 hours | Glucose at 1.5 hours |
|---|---|---|---|---|
| Breakfast |  |  |  |  |
| Snack |  |  |  |  |
| Lunch |  |  |  |  |
| Snack |  |  |  |  |
| Dinner |  |  |  |  |

STRESS LEVEL _____

Low  ——————————————————————→  High

1     2     3     4     5     6     7     8     9     10

EXERCISE   Type _____          Yes     No

MEDITATION/DEEP BREATHING                    Yes     No

VITAMIN                                       Yes     No

EIGHT GLASSES OF WATER                        Yes     No

DATE _____

MORNING BLOOD GLUCOSE _____

WEIGHT _____

CUP OF HOT WATER          Yes    No

|  | Meal | Time | Time + 1.5 hours | Glucose at 1.5 hours |
|---|---|---|---|---|
| Breakfast |  |  |  |  |
| Snack |  |  |  |  |
| Lunch |  |  |  |  |
| Snack |  |  |  |  |
| Dinner |  |  |  |  |

STRESS LEVEL _____

Low  ————————————————————————→  High

1    2    3    4    5    6    7    8    9    10

EXERCISE   Type _____          Yes    No

MEDITATION/DEEP BREATHING                        Yes    No

VITAMIN                                          Yes    No

EIGHT GLASSES OF WATER                           Yes    No

DATE _____

MORNING BLOOD GLUCOSE _____

WEIGHT _____

CUP OF HOT WATER         Yes    No

|  | Meal | Time | Time + 1.5 hours | Glucose at 1.5 hours |
|---|---|---|---|---|
| Breakfast |  |  |  |  |
| Snack |  |  |  |  |
| Lunch |  |  |  |  |
| Snack |  |  |  |  |
| Dinner |  |  |  |  |

STRESS LEVEL _____

Low ————————————————————➤ High

1    2    3    4    5    6    7    8    9    10

EXERCISE   Type _____       Yes    No

MEDITATION/DEEP BREATHING       Yes    No

VITAMIN       Yes    No

EIGHT GLASSES OF WATER       Yes    No

DATE _____

MORNING BLOOD GLUCOSE _____

WEIGHT _____

CUP OF HOT WATER      Yes   No

|  | Meal | Time | Time + 1.5 hours | Glucose at 1.5 hours |
|---|---|---|---|---|
| Breakfast |  |  |  |  |
| Snack |  |  |  |  |
| Lunch |  |  |  |  |
| Snack |  |  |  |  |
| Dinner |  |  |  |  |

STRESS LEVEL _____

Low ⟶ High

1    2    3    4    5    6    7    8    9   10

EXERCISE  Type _____    Yes    No

MEDITATION/DEEP BREATHING    Yes    No

VITAMIN    Yes    No

EIGHT GLASSES OF WATER    Yes    No

DATE _____

MORNING BLOOD GLUCOSE _____

WEIGHT _____

CUP OF HOT WATER          Yes     No

|  | Meal | Time | Time + 1.5 hours | Glucose at 1.5 hours |
|---|---|---|---|---|
| Breakfast |  |  |  |  |
| Snack |  |  |  |  |
| Lunch |  |  |  |  |
| Snack |  |  |  |  |
| Dinner |  |  |  |  |

STRESS LEVEL _____

Low ⟶ High

1     2     3     4     5     6     7     8     9     10

EXERCISE  Type _____          Yes     No

MEDITATION/DEEP BREATHING          Yes     No

VITAMIN          Yes     No

EIGHT GLASSES OF WATER          Yes     No

DATE _____

MORNING BLOOD GLUCOSE _____

WEIGHT _____

CUP OF HOT WATER          Yes     No

|  | Meal | Time | Time + 1.5 hours | Glucose at 1.5 hours |
|---|---|---|---|---|
| Breakfast |  |  |  |  |
| Snack |  |  |  |  |
| Lunch |  |  |  |  |
| Snack |  |  |  |  |
| Dinner |  |  |  |  |

STRESS LEVEL _____

Low ————————————————————➤ High

  1    2    3    4    5    6    7    8    9    10

EXERCISE   Type _____          Yes     No

MEDITATION/DEEP BREATHING                          Yes     No

VITAMIN                                            Yes     No

EIGHT GLASSES OF WATER                             Yes     No

DATE _____

MORNING BLOOD GLUCOSE _____

WEIGHT _____

CUP OF HOT WATER          Yes     No

|  | Meal | Time | Time + 1.5 hours | Glucose at 1.5 hours |
|---|---|---|---|---|
| Breakfast |  |  |  |  |
| Snack |  |  |  |  |
| Lunch |  |  |  |  |
| Snack |  |  |  |  |
| Dinner |  |  |  |  |

STRESS LEVEL _____

Low ————————————————————————➤ High

  1     2     3     4     5     6     7     8     9     10

EXERCISE   Type _____          Yes     No

MEDITATION/DEEP BREATHING                              Yes     No

VITAMIN                                                Yes     No

EIGHT GLASSES OF WATER                                 Yes     No

DATE _____

MORNING BLOOD GLUCOSE _____

WEIGHT _____

CUP OF HOT WATER          Yes     No

|  | Meal | Time | Time + 1.5 hours | Glucose at 1.5 hours |
|---|---|---|---|---|
| Breakfast |  |  |  |  |
| Snack |  |  |  |  |
| Lunch |  |  |  |  |
| Snack |  |  |  |  |
| Dinner |  |  |  |  |

STRESS LEVEL _____

Low  ———————————————————➤ High

  1      2      3      4      5      6      7      8      9      10

EXERCISE   Type _____          Yes     No

MEDITATION/DEEP BREATHING                      Yes     No

VITAMIN                                         Yes     No

EIGHT GLASSES OF WATER                          Yes     No

DATE _____

MORNING BLOOD GLUCOSE _____

WEIGHT _____

CUP OF HOT WATER          Yes    No

|  | Meal | Time | Time + 1.5 hours | Glucose at 1.5 hours |
|---|---|---|---|---|
| Breakfast |  |  |  |  |
| Snack |  |  |  |  |
| Lunch |  |  |  |  |
| Snack |  |  |  |  |
| Dinner |  |  |  |  |

STRESS LEVEL _____

Low ————————————————————→ High

1      2      3      4      5      6      7      8      9      10

EXERCISE   Type _____          Yes    No

MEDITATION/DEEP BREATHING                              Yes    No

VITAMIN                                               Yes    No

EIGHT GLASSES OF WATER                                Yes    No

DATE _____

MORNING BLOOD GLUCOSE _____

WEIGHT _____

CUP OF HOT WATER          Yes     No

| | Meal | Time | Time + 1.5 hours | Glucose at 1.5 hours |
|---|---|---|---|---|
| Breakfast | | | | |
| Snack | | | | |
| Lunch | | | | |
| Snack | | | | |
| Dinner | | | | |

STRESS LEVEL _____

Low ——————————————————➤ High

 1     2     3     4     5     6     7     8     9     10

EXERCISE   Type _____          Yes     No

MEDITATION/DEEP BREATHING                              Yes     No

VITAMIN                                                Yes     No

EIGHT GLASSES OF WATER                                 Yes     No

DATE _____

MORNING BLOOD GLUCOSE _____

WEIGHT _____

CUP OF HOT WATER          Yes     No

| | Meal | Time | Time + 1.5 hours | Glucose at 1.5 hours |
|---|---|---|---|---|
| Breakfast | | | | |
| Snack | | | | |
| Lunch | | | | |
| Snack | | | | |
| Dinner | | | | |

STRESS LEVEL _____

Low ————————————————————→ High

1      2      3      4      5      6      7      8      9      10

EXERCISE   Type _____          Yes     No

MEDITATION/DEEP BREATHING                         Yes     No

VITAMIN                                           Yes     No

EIGHT GLASSES OF WATER                            Yes     No

DATE _____

MORNING BLOOD GLUCOSE _____

WEIGHT _____

CUP OF HOT WATER          Yes     No

|  | Meal | Time | Time + 1.5 hours | Glucose at 1.5 hours |
|---|---|---|---|---|
| Breakfast |  |  |  |  |
| Snack |  |  |  |  |
| Lunch |  |  |  |  |
| Snack |  |  |  |  |
| Dinner |  |  |  |  |

STRESS LEVEL _____

Low  ————————————————→ High
  1      2      3      4      5      6      7      8      9     10

EXERCISE  Type _____          Yes     No

MEDITATION/DEEP BREATHING                        Yes     No

VITAMIN                                          Yes     No

EIGHT GLASSES OF WATER                           Yes     No

DATE _____

MORNING BLOOD GLUCOSE _____

WEIGHT _____

CUP OF HOT WATER          Yes     No

|           | Meal | Time | Time +<br>1.5 hours | Glucose at<br>1.5 hours |
|-----------|------|------|---------------------|--------------------------|
| Breakfast |      |      |                     |                          |
| Snack     |      |      |                     |                          |
| Lunch     |      |      |                     |                          |
| Snack     |      |      |                     |                          |
| Dinner    |      |      |                     |                          |

STRESS LEVEL _____

Low ————————————————————————➤ High

 1     2     3     4     5     6     7     8     9     10

EXERCISE  Type _____          Yes     No

MEDITATION/DEEP BREATHING                        Yes     No

VITAMIN                                           Yes     No

EIGHT GLASSES OF WATER                            Yes     No

DATE _____

MORNING BLOOD GLUCOSE _____

WEIGHT _____

CUP OF HOT WATER      Yes    No

|  | Meal | Time | Time + 1.5 hours | Glucose at 1.5 hours |
|---|---|---|---|---|
| Breakfast |  |  |  |  |
| Snack |  |  |  |  |
| Lunch |  |  |  |  |
| Snack |  |  |  |  |
| Dinner |  |  |  |  |

STRESS LEVEL _____

Low  ⟶  High

   1    2    3    4    5    6    7    8    9    10

EXERCISE   Type _____      Yes    No

MEDITATION/DEEP BREATHING      Yes    No

VITAMIN      Yes    No

EIGHT GLASSES OF WATER      Yes    No

DATE _____

MORNING BLOOD GLUCOSE _____

WEIGHT _____

CUP OF HOT WATER          Yes     No

| | Meal | Time | Time + 1.5 hours | Glucose at 1.5 hours |
|---|---|---|---|---|
| Breakfast | | | | |
| Snack | | | | |
| Lunch | | | | |
| Snack | | | | |
| Dinner | | | | |

STRESS LEVEL _____

Low ————————————————————→ High

1     2     3     4     5     6     7     8     9     10

EXERCISE  Type _____          Yes     No

MEDITATION/DEEP BREATHING          Yes     No

VITAMIN          Yes     No

EIGHT GLASSES OF WATER          Yes     No

DATE _____

MORNING BLOOD GLUCOSE _____

WEIGHT _____

CUP OF HOT WATER          Yes    No

|  | Meal | Time | Time + 1.5 hours | Glucose at 1.5 hours |
|---|---|---|---|---|
| Breakfast |  |  |  |  |
| Snack |  |  |  |  |
| Lunch |  |  |  |  |
| Snack |  |  |  |  |
| Dinner |  |  |  |  |

STRESS LEVEL _____

Low $\longrightarrow$ High

1     2     3     4     5     6     7     8     9     10

EXERCISE   Type _____          Yes    No

MEDITATION/DEEP BREATHING                         Yes    No

VITAMIN                                            Yes    No

EIGHT GLASSES OF WATER                            Yes    No

DATE _____

MORNING BLOOD GLUCOSE _____

WEIGHT _____

CUP OF HOT WATER          Yes     No

|  | Meal | Time | Time + 1.5 hours | Glucose at 1.5 hours |
|---|---|---|---|---|
| Breakfast |  |  |  |  |
| Snack |  |  |  |  |
| Lunch |  |  |  |  |
| Snack |  |  |  |  |
| Dinner |  |  |  |  |

STRESS LEVEL _____

Low ⟶ High

| 1 | 2 | 3 | 4 | 5 | 6 | 7 | 8 | 9 | 10 |

EXERCISE  Type _____          Yes     No

MEDITATION/DEEP BREATHING          Yes     No

VITAMIN          Yes     No

EIGHT GLASSES OF WATER          Yes     No

## LIFE GOALS . . . for the Last 4 Weeks

The simple task of listing your goals has a powerful effect on organizing your priorities and helping you to achieve your health, career and happiness desires.

1. List goals in the numbered spaces.
2. Under each goal—list three action steps necessary on YOUR part to achieve the written goal.
3. Once an action step or a goal is achieved, cross it off with a red pen.

GOAL 1: _____

    Action Step A: _____

    Action Step B: _____

    Action Step C: _____

GOAL 2: _____

    Action Step A: _____

    Action Step B: _____

    Action Step C: _____

GOAL 3: _____

    Action Step A: _____

    Action Step B: _____

    Action Step C: _____

GOAL 4: _____

    Action Step A: _____

    Action Step B: _____

    Action Step C: _____

GOAL 5: _____

    Action Step A: _____

    Action Step B: _____

    Action Step C: _____

GOAL 6: _____

    Action Step A: _____

    Action Step B: _____

    Action Step C: _____

GOAL 7: _____

    Action Step A: _____

    Action Step B: _____

    Action Step C: _____

DATE _____

MORNING BLOOD GLUCOSE _____

WEIGHT _____

CUP OF HOT WATER          Yes     No

| | Meal | Time | Time + 1.5 hours | Glucose at 1.5 hours |
|---|---|---|---|---|
| Breakfast | | | | |
| Snack | | | | |
| Lunch | | | | |
| Snack | | | | |
| Dinner | | | | |

STRESS LEVEL _____

Low ————————————————————➤ High
  1     2     3     4     5     6     7     8     9     10

EXERCISE   Type _____          Yes     No

MEDITATION/DEEP BREATHING                         Yes     No

VITAMIN                                           Yes     No

EIGHT GLASSES OF WATER                            Yes     No

DATE _____

MORNING BLOOD GLUCOSE _____

WEIGHT _____

CUP OF HOT WATER          Yes     No

|  | Meal | Time | Time + 1.5 hours | Glucose at 1.5 hours |
|---|---|---|---|---|
| Breakfast |  |  |  |  |
| Snack |  |  |  |  |
| Lunch |  |  |  |  |
| Snack |  |  |  |  |
| Dinner |  |  |  |  |

STRESS LEVEL _____

Low  ————————————————————————➤  High
  1      2      3      4      5      6      7      8      9     10

EXERCISE   Type _____          Yes     No

MEDITATION/DEEP BREATHING                        Yes     No

VITAMIN                                          Yes     No

EIGHT GLASSES OF WATER                           Yes     No

DATE _____

MORNING BLOOD GLUCOSE _____

WEIGHT _____

CUP OF HOT WATER          Yes     No

|  | Meal | Time | Time + 1.5 hours | Glucose at 1.5 hours |
|---|---|---|---|---|
| Breakfast |  |  |  |  |
| Snack |  |  |  |  |
| Lunch |  |  |  |  |
| Snack |  |  |  |  |
| Dinner |  |  |  |  |

STRESS LEVEL _____

Low ————————————————→ High

1     2     3     4     5     6     7     8     9     10

EXERCISE   Type _____          Yes     No

MEDITATION/DEEP BREATHING                        Yes     No

VITAMIN                                          Yes     No

EIGHT GLASSES OF WATER                           Yes     No

DATE _____

MORNING BLOOD GLUCOSE _____

WEIGHT _____

CUP OF HOT WATER      Yes    No

| | Meal | Time | Time + 1.5 hours | Glucose at 1.5 hours |
|---|---|---|---|---|
| Breakfast | | | | |
| Snack | | | | |
| Lunch | | | | |
| Snack | | | | |
| Dinner | | | | |

STRESS LEVEL _____

Low ————————————————▶ High

1    2    3    4    5    6    7    8    9    10

EXERCISE   Type _____      Yes    No

MEDITATION/DEEP BREATHING                      Yes    No

VITAMIN                                        Yes    No

EIGHT GLASSES OF WATER                         Yes    No

DATE _____

MORNING BLOOD GLUCOSE _____

WEIGHT _____

CUP OF HOT WATER        Yes     No

|  | Meal | Time | Time + 1.5 hours | Glucose at 1.5 hours |
|---|---|---|---|---|
| Breakfast |  |  |  |  |
| Snack |  |  |  |  |
| Lunch |  |  |  |  |
| Snack |  |  |  |  |
| Dinner |  |  |  |  |

STRESS LEVEL _____

Low $\longrightarrow$ High

1     2     3     4     5     6     7     8     9     10

EXERCISE   Type _____        Yes     No

MEDITATION/DEEP BREATHING                              Yes     No

VITAMIN                                                                    Yes     No

EIGHT GLASSES OF WATER                                   Yes     No

DATE _____

MORNING BLOOD GLUCOSE _____

WEIGHT _____

CUP OF HOT WATER          Yes     No

|  | Meal | Time | Time + 1.5 hours | Glucose at 1.5 hours |
|---|---|---|---|---|
| Breakfast |  |  |  |  |
| Snack |  |  |  |  |
| Lunch |  |  |  |  |
| Snack |  |  |  |  |
| Dinner |  |  |  |  |

STRESS LEVEL _____

Low ————————————————————➤ High

1      2      3      4      5      6      7      8      9      10

EXERCISE   Type _____          Yes     No

MEDITATION/DEEP BREATHING                          Yes     No

VITAMIN                                             Yes     No

EIGHT GLASSES OF WATER                             Yes     No

DATE _____

MORNING BLOOD GLUCOSE _____

WEIGHT _____

CUP OF HOT WATER          Yes     No

|  | Meal | Time | Time + 1.5 hours | Glucose at 1.5 hours |
|---|---|---|---|---|
| Breakfast |  |  |  |  |
| Snack |  |  |  |  |
| Lunch |  |  |  |  |
| Snack |  |  |  |  |
| Dinner |  |  |  |  |

STRESS LEVEL _____

Low ————————————————→ High

1     2     3     4     5     6     7     8     9     10

EXERCISE   Type _____          Yes     No

MEDITATION/DEEP BREATHING          Yes     No

VITAMIN          Yes     No

EIGHT GLASSES OF WATER          Yes     No

DATE _____

MORNING BLOOD GLUCOSE _____

WEIGHT _____

CUP OF HOT WATER          Yes     No

| | Meal | Time | Time + 1.5 hours | Glucose at 1.5 hours |
|---|---|---|---|---|
| Breakfast | | | | |
| Snack | | | | |
| Lunch | | | | |
| Snack | | | | |
| Dinner | | | | |

STRESS LEVEL _____

Low ————————————————————→ High

| 1 | 2 | 3 | 4 | 5 | 6 | 7 | 8 | 9 | 10 |
|---|---|---|---|---|---|---|---|---|---|

EXERCISE  Type _____          Yes     No

MEDITATION/DEEP BREATHING          Yes     No

VITAMIN          Yes     No

EIGHT GLASSES OF WATER          Yes     No

DATE _____

MORNING BLOOD GLUCOSE _____

WEIGHT _____

CUP OF HOT WATER          Yes     No

|  | Meal | Time | Time + 1.5 hours | Glucose at 1.5 hours |
|---|---|---|---|---|
| Breakfast |  |  |  |  |
| Snack |  |  |  |  |
| Lunch |  |  |  |  |
| Snack |  |  |  |  |
| Dinner |  |  |  |  |

STRESS LEVEL _____

Low ————————————————————→ High

  1     2     3     4     5     6     7     8     9     10

EXERCISE   Type _____          Yes     No

MEDITATION/DEEP BREATHING                                  Yes     No

VITAMIN                                                             Yes     No

EIGHT GLASSES OF WATER                                      Yes     No

DATE _____

MORNING BLOOD GLUCOSE _____

WEIGHT _____

CUP OF HOT WATER          Yes     No

| | Meal | Time | Time + 1.5 hours | Glucose at 1.5 hours |
|---|---|---|---|---|
| Breakfast | | | | |
| Snack | | | | |
| Lunch | | | | |
| Snack | | | | |
| Dinner | | | | |

STRESS LEVEL _____

Low ⟶ High

1     2     3     4     5     6     7     8     9     10

EXERCISE   Type _____          Yes     No

MEDITATION/DEEP BREATHING                              Yes     No

VITAMIN                                                Yes     No

EIGHT GLASSES OF WATER                                 Yes     No

DATE _____

MORNING BLOOD GLUCOSE _____

WEIGHT _____

CUP OF HOT WATER          Yes    No

|  | Meal | Time | Time + 1.5 hours | Glucose at 1.5 hours |
|---|---|---|---|---|
| Breakfast |  |  |  |  |
| Snack |  |  |  |  |
| Lunch |  |  |  |  |
| Snack |  |  |  |  |
| Dinner |  |  |  |  |

STRESS LEVEL _____

Low ——————————————————→ High

1    2    3    4    5    6    7    8    9    10

EXERCISE   Type _____          Yes    No

MEDITATION/DEEP BREATHING                              Yes    No

VITAMIN                                                Yes    No

EIGHT GLASSES OF WATER                                Yes    No

DATE _____

MORNING BLOOD GLUCOSE _____

WEIGHT _____

CUP OF HOT WATER     Yes    No

| | Meal | Time | Time + 1.5 hours | Glucose at 1.5 hours |
|---|---|---|---|---|
| Breakfast | | | | |
| Snack | | | | |
| Lunch | | | | |
| Snack | | | | |
| Dinner | | | | |

STRESS LEVEL _____

Low ⟶ High

1     2     3     4     5     6     7     8     9     10

EXERCISE  Type _____          Yes     No

MEDITATION/DEEP BREATHING                       Yes     No

VITAMIN                                          Yes     No

EIGHT GLASSES OF WATER                           Yes     No

DATE _____

MORNING BLOOD GLUCOSE _____

WEIGHT _____

CUP OF HOT WATER        Yes    No

| | Meal | Time | Time + 1.5 hours | Glucose at 1.5 hours |
|---|---|---|---|---|
| Breakfast | | | | |
| Snack | | | | |
| Lunch | | | | |
| Snack | | | | |
| Dinner | | | | |

STRESS LEVEL _____

Low ————————————————▶ High

  1     2     3     4     5     6     7     8     9     10

EXERCISE  Type _____        Yes    No

MEDITATION/DEEP BREATHING                          Yes    No

VITAMIN                                            Yes    No

EIGHT GLASSES OF WATER                             Yes    No

DATE _____

MORNING BLOOD GLUCOSE _____

WEIGHT _____

CUP OF HOT WATER          Yes     No

|  | Meal | Time | Time + 1.5 hours | Glucose at 1.5 hours |
|---|---|---|---|---|
| Breakfast |  |  |  |  |
| Snack |  |  |  |  |
| Lunch |  |  |  |  |
| Snack |  |  |  |  |
| Dinner |  |  |  |  |

STRESS LEVEL _____

Low ———————————————————→ High

1     2     3     4     5     6     7     8     9     10

EXERCISE   Type _____          Yes     No

MEDITATION/DEEP BREATHING                          Yes     No

VITAMIN                                            Yes     No

EIGHT GLASSES OF WATER                             Yes     No

DATE _____

MORNING BLOOD GLUCOSE _____

WEIGHT _____

CUP OF HOT WATER          Yes     No

| | Meal | Time | Time + 1.5 hours | Glucose at 1.5 hours |
|---|---|---|---|---|
| Breakfast | | | | |
| Snack | | | | |
| Lunch | | | | |
| Snack | | | | |
| Dinner | | | | |

STRESS LEVEL _____

Low ⟶ High

| 1 | 2 | 3 | 4 | 5 | 6 | 7 | 8 | 9 | 10 |

EXERCISE   Type _____          Yes     No

MEDITATION/DEEP BREATHING          Yes     No

VITAMIN          Yes     No

EIGHT GLASSES OF WATER          Yes     No

DATE _____

MORNING BLOOD GLUCOSE _____

WEIGHT _____

CUP OF HOT WATER          Yes     No

|  | Meal | Time | Time + 1.5 hours | Glucose at 1.5 hours |
|---|---|---|---|---|
| Breakfast |  |  |  |  |
| Snack |  |  |  |  |
| Lunch |  |  |  |  |
| Snack |  |  |  |  |
| Dinner |  |  |  |  |

STRESS LEVEL _____

Low ————————————————————→ High

1     2     3     4     5     6     7     8     9     10

EXERCISE   Type _____          Yes     No

MEDITATION/DEEP BREATHING                          Yes     No

VITAMIN                                            Yes     No

EIGHT GLASSES OF WATER                             Yes     No

DATE _____

MORNING BLOOD GLUCOSE _____

WEIGHT _____

CUP OF HOT WATER        Yes    No

|  | Meal | Time | Time + 1.5 hours | Glucose at 1.5 hours |
|---|---|---|---|---|
| Breakfast |  |  |  |  |
| Snack |  |  |  |  |
| Lunch |  |  |  |  |
| Snack |  |  |  |  |
| Dinner |  |  |  |  |

STRESS LEVEL _____

Low ————————————————————→ High

  1    2    3    4    5    6    7    8    9   10

EXERCISE   Type _____        Yes    No

MEDITATION/DEEP BREATHING                         Yes    No

VITAMIN                                                          Yes    No

EIGHT GLASSES OF WATER                             Yes    No

DATE _____

MORNING BLOOD GLUCOSE _____

WEIGHT _____

CUP OF HOT WATER          Yes     No

|  | Meal | Time | Time + 1.5 hours | Glucose at 1.5 hours |
|---|---|---|---|---|
| Breakfast |  |  |  |  |
| Snack |  |  |  |  |
| Lunch |  |  |  |  |
| Snack |  |  |  |  |
| Dinner |  |  |  |  |

STRESS LEVEL _____

Low ⟶ High

1     2     3     4     5     6     7     8     9     10

EXERCISE  Type _____          Yes     No

MEDITATION/DEEP BREATHING          Yes     No

VITAMIN          Yes     No

EIGHT GLASSES OF WATER          Yes     No

DATE  _____

MORNING BLOOD GLUCOSE  _____

WEIGHT  _____

CUP OF HOT WATER          Yes     No

|  | Meal | Time | Time + 1.5 hours | Glucose at 1.5 hours |
|---|---|---|---|---|
| Breakfast |  |  |  |  |
| Snack |  |  |  |  |
| Lunch |  |  |  |  |
| Snack |  |  |  |  |
| Dinner |  |  |  |  |

STRESS LEVEL  _____

Low ⟶ High

1     2     3     4     5     6     7     8     9     10

EXERCISE   Type _____          Yes     No

MEDITATION/DEEP BREATHING                    Yes     No

VITAMIN                                       Yes     No

EIGHT GLASSES OF WATER                        Yes     No

DATE _____

MORNING BLOOD GLUCOSE _____

WEIGHT _____

CUP OF HOT WATER          Yes     No

|  | Meal | Time | Time + 1.5 hours | Glucose at 1.5 hours |
|---|---|---|---|---|
| Breakfast |  |  |  |  |
| Snack |  |  |  |  |
| Lunch |  |  |  |  |
| Snack |  |  |  |  |
| Dinner |  |  |  |  |

STRESS LEVEL _____

Low ——————————————→ High
1     2     3     4     5     6     7     8     9     10

EXERCISE   Type _____          Yes     No

MEDITATION/DEEP BREATHING                          Yes     No

VITAMIN                                            Yes     No

EIGHT GLASSES OF WATER                             Yes     No

DATE _____

MORNING BLOOD GLUCOSE _____

WEIGHT _____

CUP OF HOT WATER          Yes    No

| | Meal | Time | Time + 1.5 hours | Glucose at 1.5 hours |
|---|---|---|---|---|
| Breakfast | | | | |
| Snack | | | | |
| Lunch | | | | |
| Snack | | | | |
| Dinner | | | | |

STRESS LEVEL _____

Low ⟶ High

1    2    3    4    5    6    7    8    9    10

EXERCISE   Type _____          Yes    No

MEDITATION/DEEP BREATHING                Yes    No

VITAMIN                                  Yes    No

EIGHT GLASSES OF WATER                   Yes    No

DATE _____

MORNING BLOOD GLUCOSE _____

WEIGHT _____

CUP OF HOT WATER          Yes     No

|  | Meal | Time | Time + 1.5 hours | Glucose at 1.5 hours |
|---|---|---|---|---|
| Breakfast |  |  |  |  |
| Snack |  |  |  |  |
| Lunch |  |  |  |  |
| Snack |  |  |  |  |
| Dinner |  |  |  |  |

STRESS LEVEL _____

Low ——————————————————————➤ High

1      2      3      4      5      6      7      8      9      10

EXERCISE  Type _____          Yes     No

MEDITATION/DEEP BREATHING                          Yes     No

VITAMIN                                             Yes     No

EIGHT GLASSES OF WATER                             Yes     No

DATE _____

MORNING BLOOD GLUCOSE _____

WEIGHT _____

CUP OF HOT WATER　　　Yes　　No

|  | Meal | Time | Time + 1.5 hours | Glucose at 1.5 hours |
|---|---|---|---|---|
| Breakfast |  |  |  |  |
| Snack |  |  |  |  |
| Lunch |  |  |  |  |
| Snack |  |  |  |  |
| Dinner |  |  |  |  |

STRESS LEVEL _____

Low ⟶ High

　1　　2　　3　　4　　5　　6　　7　　8　　9　　10

EXERCISE　Type _____　　Yes　　No

MEDITATION/DEEP BREATHING　　　　　　Yes　　No

VITAMIN　　　　　　　　　　　　　　　Yes　　No

EIGHT GLASSES OF WATER　　　　　　　　Yes　　No

DATE _____

MORNING BLOOD GLUCOSE _____

WEIGHT _____

CUP OF HOT WATER          Yes    No

|  | Meal | Time | Time + 1.5 hours | Glucose at 1.5 hours |
|---|---|---|---|---|
| Breakfast |  |  |  |  |
| Snack |  |  |  |  |
| Lunch |  |  |  |  |
| Snack |  |  |  |  |
| Dinner |  |  |  |  |

STRESS LEVEL _____

Low ————————————————→ High

1     2     3     4     5     6     7     8     9     10

EXERCISE   Type _____          Yes     No

MEDITATION/DEEP BREATHING                  Yes     No

VITAMIN                                     Yes     No

EIGHT GLASSES OF WATER                      Yes     No

DATE _____

MORNING BLOOD GLUCOSE _____

WEIGHT _____

CUP OF HOT WATER          Yes     No

|  | Meal | Time | Time + 1.5 hours | Glucose at 1.5 hours |
|---|---|---|---|---|
| Breakfast |  |  |  |  |
| Snack |  |  |  |  |
| Lunch |  |  |  |  |
| Snack |  |  |  |  |
| Dinner |  |  |  |  |

STRESS LEVEL _____

Low ⟶ High

1     2     3     4     5     6     7     8     9     10

EXERCISE   Type _____          Yes     No

MEDITATION/DEEP BREATHING                        Yes     No

VITAMIN                                          Yes     No

EIGHT GLASSES OF WATER                           Yes     No

DATE _____

MORNING BLOOD GLUCOSE _____

WEIGHT _____

CUP OF HOT WATER          Yes    No

|  | Meal | Time | Time + 1.5 hours | Glucose at 1.5 hours |
|---|---|---|---|---|
| Breakfast |  |  |  |  |
| Snack |  |  |  |  |
| Lunch |  |  |  |  |
| Snack |  |  |  |  |
| Dinner |  |  |  |  |

STRESS LEVEL _____

Low ──────────────────────────▶ High

1    2    3    4    5    6    7    8    9    10

EXERCISE   Type _____          Yes    No

MEDITATION/DEEP BREATHING          Yes    No

VITAMIN          Yes    No

EIGHT GLASSES OF WATER          Yes    No

DATE _____

MORNING BLOOD GLUCOSE _____

WEIGHT _____

CUP OF HOT WATER          Yes     No

| | Meal | Time | Time + 1.5 hours | Glucose at 1.5 hours |
|---|---|---|---|---|
| Breakfast | | | | |
| Snack | | | | |
| Lunch | | | | |
| Snack | | | | |
| Dinner | | | | |

STRESS LEVEL _____

Low  ⟶  High

1     2     3     4     5     6     7     8     9     10

EXERCISE   Type _____          Yes     No

MEDITATION/DEEP BREATHING                    Yes     No

VITAMIN                                       Yes     No

EIGHT GLASSES OF WATER                        Yes     No

DATE _____

MORNING BLOOD GLUCOSE _____

WEIGHT _____

CUP OF HOT WATER      Yes    No

| | Meal | Time | Time + 1.5 hours | Glucose at 1.5 hours |
|---|---|---|---|---|
| Breakfast | | | | |
| Snack | | | | |
| Lunch | | | | |
| Snack | | | | |
| Dinner | | | | |

STRESS LEVEL _____

Low ⟶ High

1    2    3    4    5    6    7    8    9    10

EXERCISE   Type _____        Yes    No

MEDITATION/DEEP BREATHING                      Yes    No

VITAMIN                                         Yes    No

EIGHT GLASSES OF WATER                          Yes    No

## Testimonials

> *Every human being is the author of*
> *his own health or disease.*
> *—Buddha*

*"I followed Candice's diet plan one year ago. I was 45 pounds overweight with high blood pressure, a cholesterol problem and Type 2 diabetes. I took off 35 pounds in the eight-week period and continued with another 20 over the year. At a checkup in April, my cholesterol was way down, I was taken off the blood pressure medication and the Metformin for diabetes.*

*"The weight has stayed off. The eating pattern becomes a way of life. My sugar levels are rarely above 100.*

*"I do test every morning. I will also, at this point, eat whatever I want when out or at a party and try to keep it in line the next day. This diet changed my life. I think it is successful because of the immediate reinforcement of testing . . . You are in charge of what goes in your mouth and you can see the result immediately."*

—SALLY P.

*"I love working with Candice and I love the diet! Before starting the Pancreatic Nutritional Program, I ate all day. There was no structure to my eating. The PNP gave me definition. I now have three meals a day and I love the way I'm eating. I haven't been perfect. I still have some sugar, some alcohol and cream in the occasional cup of coffee. However, I do so now in moderation and I'm still losing weight even though I haven't been totally*

*strict on the program. I have given up most meat. Eliminating a good portion of the animal products in my diet has made me feel really great. After 12 weeks on the PNP, my blood work improved significantly. My triglycerides and overall cholesterol went down quite a bit. I lost 23 pounds and I've signed up for another 12 weeks in order to lose 10–15 more. Prior to meeting with Candice, I had recently developed chin acne and was about to see a dermatologist about getting a prescription to clear it up. Candice asked me to hold off and see if the diet she was advocating would have a positive effect. Well, my skin looks so much better after 12 weeks on the PNP. It looks much younger and clearer. Friends and family notice, too. I am very grateful for the PNP, for Candice's counseling and the change both have made in my life."*     —K. S.

*"Candice Rosen and* The Pancreatic Oath *changed my life . . . After doing the PNP for eight weeks I felt 10 years younger . . . I had so much energy and felt wonderful . . . I lost 15 pounds in the eight weeks . . . it is still off, over a year later . . . This is the only way to live . . . I highly recommend it to everyone."*     — GINNA B.

*"I followed Candice Rosen's weight loss plan and lost 20 pounds in six weeks! I didn't find it very difficult, just a little discipline, and boy, do those pounds fall off. It becomes a way of eating rather than a diet."*     —YALE S.

*"I came to the Pancreatic Nutritional Program through a referral. My co-worker who was overweight, depressed, and low energy*

*was now getting skinny and full of pep. Her outlook on life was even improving. I had to know her secret. She said it was the PNP!*

*"However, at first, I didn't think it was something that could help me. I was not only overweight and tired, but I was also suffering from Type 2 diabetes and rheumatoid arthritis. When I began my counseling sessions, I didn't really believe in my own ability to impact my health. I couldn't control my emotional eating. I had no understanding of the biology behind my cravings.*

*"After losing 46 lbs, getting off my medications . . . and finally putting on a bathing suit this vacation (after 15 years of t-shirts and shorts at the beach), I'm a believer! I am in less pain from my arthritis and have even started a low impact exercise routine. My daughters (13 and 19) have now entered the Family Counseling program and they are improving their health, too, by learning how to eat better. I don't want them to suffer as I have over the years. I don't want them to ever resort to yo-yo dieting. The PNP has given us a new outlook on life. I am forever grateful to Candice!"*

—Maria A.

*"I am a marathon runner and an avid cyclist. Even though I was active and the picture of health, inside I was the opposite. I had alarmingly high cholesterol and triglycerides. I thought I was eating healthy and nourishing by body properly. However, at my annual physical I was told I needed to be on a statin drug. I was beyond confused. My partner told me about the PNP. I entered the program and it changed my life. No medication. No more caffeine addiction. No more headaches. Best part, I now sleep through the night. Thank you, Candice!"* —Bruce W.

*"I was diagnosed at 24 with polycystic ovarian syndrome (PCOS). My symptoms included irregular periods, embarrassing body hair, acne, and a spare tire around my middle. Working with my endocrinologist, my gynecologist, and the registered dietician at the hospital had not made a dent in my symptoms. After entering the Pancreatic Nutritional Program . . . I became hooked on learning more about my body and how simple changes could have a major impact on my health over time. I am mid-way through the PNP Detox now, and I use the tools provided to tweak my diet in order to manage my condition. Instead of trying to mask my symptoms with different medications, I got to the cause of them . . . I look hot and, more importantly, I feel hot. Finally losing the freshman 15 that stayed on since college."*

—LETESHA J.

*"Today is the end of 12 weeks. You told me I would lose between 20 and 31 pounds. I ended up at exactly minus 25 pounds . . . Please sign me up for another 12 weeks . . . I was at a wedding with {name removed} and found out she is on the PNP, too! She looks great."* —AL F.

*"When I first began working with Candice and the Pancreatic Nutritional Program I weighed 260 pounds and stood at 5'9". I had horrible eating habits that included eating out for at least one meal of the day, drinking a sugar-filled espresso drink from Starbucks on a daily basis, as well as an addiction to Diet Coke that consisted of at least three Diet Cokes a day. What I find so wonderful about this program is that once you learn the basics of it you can continue with it on your own. The PNP does not*

*have you eat 'their specific food' nor does it require you to count anything—be it calories or points. With the help and instruction of Candice, I was able to lose 25 pounds in eight weeks. I have continued to lose 10 more pounds bringing my total weight down to 225. What I am most grateful for is learning how to look at food and where it belongs in my life. Prior to working with Candice, this was unfortunately not a top priority. I have learned that food is not my main priority and as a result have a much healthier relationship with food as well as its role in my life."*

—ALEX F., AGE 26

*"When I began my journey on the Pancreatic Nutritional Program, I was in a great deal of pain from a back injury. I had two shoulder surgeries in two years. I was a mess. I had been over 200 pounds for more than 20 years. I stood in front of Candice at 230 pounds After that, I did whatever Candice told me to do. I had tried everything under the sun and never lost more than 30 pounds. On some programs, I had even gained weight.*

*"I knew from that morning my life was going to change. Was I hungry? HELL yes, I was, but I felt great. WHY? Because I began to have feelings again. I was no longer clouded by sugar and overeating. I joined a health club. I not only exercised, but I steamed, relaxed, and learned to be quiet. I did small things every day to reward myself. Good books and music. I took Jazz 101 and loved it.*

*"I told my family to feed themselves. Two grown men . . . I thought they could handle that and they did. It took some time, but they also supported my new way of life. My son even likes*

some of my dinners and joins in. It hasn't been a year yet and I've lost over 75 pounds. I went from a size 20 to size 8 pants! Working out has reshaped my legs and arms. Also, it helped my overall mental health.

"What was so different from all the other programs I tried the meter (glucometer). The meter was the MAIN KEY! Numbers don't lie. I followed the guidelines of the PNP. What I found out was I was eating all the wrong things. That is why nothing ever worked for me. What the meter taught me was that only I could tell myself . . . what to eat and when to eat.

"I don't like to stuff food in my mouth first thing in the morning. When I was younger, I was skinny, until I had children. I never ate a meal until lunch. When I was on all those other programs, it was Eat! Eat in the morning! Eat! Eat! Eat! You know what all that eating got me in the morning? It just made me want to eat all day long! Now I enjoy hot coffee, then some tea and maybe ¼ of a pear or some nuts in the morning. I don't need that much to get me going.

"I'm 51 and the older I get, the less I need to eat. I've learned also about working out. I was overworking out with a trainer before the PNP. I needed to listen to my body and myself about workouts just like I was doing with my food. More yoga and pool. Less running and lifting.

"Those of us who have struggled with weight loss . . . we are the best excuse-makers in the world. We are better than addicts, or the most cunning of crack heads. We are junkies! Numbers became my life! No more lies to myself.

*"Pictures tell a thousand words. Once I saw the pictures of myself at a school reunion . . . I saw myself as everyone else saw me. I was FAT—HUGE at 5'3" and 230 pounds! I looked like a round ball.*

*"I no longer feel like a round ball or move like one. My life has changed so much because of the PNP. The meter was the key to the food. Most helpful for me were all my one-on-one sessions with Candice. I would have never been able to do all this on my own without Candice. Yes, it was therapy for me. I needed her more than I needed anyone. Her brown eyes were my lifeline for weeks! I never wanted to miss our sessions. I was getting stronger with every session . . . more confident with every pound lost and every weekly meeting . . . learning more about food and then about myself . . . holding that mirror up every day works for me in more ways than one!*

*"I looked at myself naked that first night I came home from Candice's office and do so every day, because it was and continues to be the naked truth! Candice maintains: The mirror doesn't lie. The scale doesn't lie. The meter doesn't lie. I stopped lying to myself. I look in the mirror every day, I weigh myself every day and I still test every day. It keeps me honest with myself. I will forever be indebted to Candice and the Pancreatic Nutritional Program for helping me find 'My Keys' so I could start the ride of my life."*

−P. HALL

## My Testimonial

What changes have you witnessed in your eating, your weight, blood work and health in the past 12 weeks? Reflect and journal it.

_____

_____

_____

_____

_____

_____

_____

_____

_____

_____

_____

_____

_____

—_____

We love to know your progress! E-mail a copy of your testimonial to info@pnprogram.com.

## Gratitude

*Feeling gratitude and not expressing it is like wrapping a present and not giving it.*
—*William Arthur Ward*

Congratulations! You have just spent the past 12 weeks protecting your pancreas by listening and responding to your body. The Pancreatic Oath: The Measurable Approach to Improved Health and Weight Loss along with The Pancreatic Oath Journal has provided you with the data you need to make wise choices about what you eat and drink, what exercise works best for you, and how stress can affect you and your blood sugar.

You, like many successful clients have a road map that illustrates the route you must travel to ensure improved health and weight loss. You may navigate off your route now and then; however, your journal and meal cards will put you back on course. Remember, your every day practice of Self Health is your lifestyle. Now that you know what is toxic for your body and your health, you can not in good conscious return to your former way of living. Be kind to yourself, protect your pancreas and celebrate health! Best Wishes, Candice Rosen

I am grateful for _____

_____

I am grateful for _____

_____

I am grateful for _____

_____

I am grateful for _____

_____

I am grateful for _____

_____

I am grateful for _____

_____

I am grateful for _____

_____

I am grateful for _____

_____

I am grateful for _____

_____

I am grateful for _____

_____

Praise yourself for having the courage to change and the fortitude to pursue your path towards optimal health. There is no going back from this point forward. You have learned the foods, combinations and portion sizes that work best for your unique body. You understand the significant role *YOU* play in your health. Your lifestyle is the practice of SELF-HEALTH. Because of the positive changes you have made with your own health and well being, you are an inspiration to your friends, family and community! Use your energy, knowledge and improved health to make a difference in the world!

## PNP™ Meal Discovery Cards

The first page provides an example of how to fill out the PNP Meal Discovery Cards. Make copies of the second page or purchase index cards to keep in a recipe holder. You will use them to record meals that work (and don't work) for your body.

Pancreas-friendly meals keep your blood glucose between: 70–100. For Diabetics, the goal is 80–140.

A meal that raises your blood glucose over 140 should never be a part of your regular diet.

The cards should serve as quick tools to help you in your meal planning.

## MY PNP™ MEAL DISCOVERY CARD

Date ___7/4___ Pancreas Friendly____ NOT ✓___

Breakfast ____ Lunch ____ Dinner ✓ Snack ____

Meal _Fried chicken, macaroni salad, potato,_
_cole slaw, soda_

_____ Glucose _196_

---

## MY PNP™ MEAL DISCOVERY CARD

Date _8/10_ Pancreas Friendly ✓__ NOT____

Breakfast ____ Lunch ✓ Dinner ____ Snack ____

Meal _Romaine and mixed green salad, oil &_
_vinegar dressing with boiled salmon, sparkling_
_water_ Glucose _88_

---

## MY PNP™ MEAL DISCOVERY CARD

Date _9/20_ Pancreas Friendly ✓__ NOT____

Breakfast ✓ Lunch ____ Dinner ____ Snack ____

Meal _Tofu scramble with vegetables, green tea_

_____ Glucose _80_

MY PNP™ MEAL DISCOVERY CARD

Date _____ Pancreas Friendly_____ NOT_____

Breakfast _____ Lunch _____ Dinner _____ Snack _____

Meal _____

_____

_____ Glucose _____

---

MY PNP™ MEAL DISCOVERY CARD

Date _____ Pancreas Friendly_____ NOT_____

Breakfast _____ Lunch _____ Dinner _____ Snack _____

Meal _____

_____

_____ Glucose _____

---

MY PNP™ MEAL DISCOVERY CARD

Date _____ Pancreas Friendly_____ NOT_____

Breakfast _____ Lunch _____ Dinner _____ Snack _____

Meal _____

_____

_____ Glucose _____

MY PNP™ MEAL DISCOVERY CARD

Date _____ Pancreas Friendly_____ NOT_____

Breakfast _____ Lunch _____ Dinner _____ Snack _____

Meal _____

_____

_____ Glucose _____

---

MY PNP™ MEAL DISCOVERY CARD

Date _____ Pancreas Friendly_____ NOT_____

Breakfast _____ Lunch _____ Dinner _____ Snack _____

Meal _____

_____

_____ Glucose _____

---

MY PNP™ MEAL DISCOVERY CARD

Date _____ Pancreas Friendly_____ NOT_____

Breakfast _____ Lunch _____ Dinner _____ Snack _____

Meal _____

_____

_____ Glucose _____

## MY PNP™ MEAL DISCOVERY CARD

Date _____ Pancreas Friendly_____ NOT_____

Breakfast _____ Lunch _____ Dinner _____ Snack _____

Meal _____

_____

_____ Glucose _____

## MY PNP™ MEAL DISCOVERY CARD

Date _____ Pancreas Friendly_____ NOT_____

Breakfast _____ Lunch _____ Dinner _____ Snack _____

Meal _____

_____

_____ Glucose _____

## MY PNP™ MEAL DISCOVERY CARD

Date _____ Pancreas Friendly_____ NOT_____

Breakfast _____ Lunch _____ Dinner _____ Snack _____

Meal _____

_____

_____ Glucose _____

MY PNP™ MEAL DISCOVERY CARD

Date _____ Pancreas Friendly____ NOT____

Breakfast ____ Lunch ____ Dinner ____ Snack ____

Meal _____

_____

_____ Glucose _____

---

MY PNP™ MEAL DISCOVERY CARD

Date _____ Pancreas Friendly____ NOT____

Breakfast ____ Lunch ____ Dinner ____ Snack ____

Meal _____

_____

_____ Glucose _____

---

MY PNP™ MEAL DISCOVERY CARD

Date _____ Pancreas Friendly____ NOT____

Breakfast ____ Lunch ____ Dinner ____ Snack ____

Meal _____

_____

_____ Glucose _____

## MY PNP™ MEAL DISCOVERY CARD

Date _____ Pancreas Friendly_____ NOT_____

Breakfast _____ Lunch _____ Dinner _____ Snack _____

Meal _____

_____

_____ Glucose _____

## MY PNP™ MEAL DISCOVERY CARD

Date _____ Pancreas Friendly_____ NOT_____

Breakfast _____ Lunch _____ Dinner _____ Snack _____

Meal _____

_____

_____ Glucose _____

## MY PNP™ MEAL DISCOVERY CARD

Date _____ Pancreas Friendly_____ NOT_____

Breakfast _____ Lunch _____ Dinner _____ Snack _____

Meal _____

_____

_____ Glucose _____

MY PNP™ MEAL DISCOVERY CARD

Date _____ Pancreas Friendly____ NOT____

Breakfast ____ Lunch ____ Dinner ____ Snack ____

Meal _____

_____

_____ Glucose ____

---

MY PNP™ MEAL DISCOVERY CARD

Date _____ Pancreas Friendly____ NOT____

Breakfast ____ Lunch ____ Dinner ____ Snack ____

Meal _____

_____

_____ Glucose ____

---

MY PNP™ MEAL DISCOVERY CARD

Date _____ Pancreas Friendly____ NOT____

Breakfast ____ Lunch ____ Dinner ____ Snack ____

Meal _____

_____

_____ Glucose ____

MY PNP™ MEAL DISCOVERY CARD

Date _____ Pancreas Friendly_____ NOT_____

Breakfast _____ Lunch _____ Dinner _____ Snack _____

Meal _____

_____

_____ Glucose _____

MY PNP™ MEAL DISCOVERY CARD

Date _____ Pancreas Friendly_____ NOT_____

Breakfast _____ Lunch _____ Dinner _____ Snack _____

Meal _____

_____

_____ Glucose _____

MY PNP™ MEAL DISCOVERY CARD

Date _____ Pancreas Friendly_____ NOT_____

Breakfast _____ Lunch _____ Dinner _____ Snack _____

Meal _____

_____

_____ Glucose _____

MY PNP™ MEAL DISCOVERY CARD

Date _____ Pancreas Friendly_____ NOT_____

Breakfast _____ Lunch _____ Dinner _____ Snack _____

Meal _____

_____

_____  Glucose _____

MY PNP™ MEAL DISCOVERY CARD

Date _____ Pancreas Friendly_____ NOT_____

Breakfast _____ Lunch _____ Dinner _____ Snack _____

Meal _____

_____

_____  Glucose _____

MY PNP™ MEAL DISCOVERY CARD

Date _____ Pancreas Friendly_____ NOT_____

Breakfast _____ Lunch _____ Dinner _____ Snack _____

Meal _____

_____

_____  Glucose _____

MY PNP™ MEAL DISCOVERY CARD

Date _____ Pancreas Friendly_____ NOT_____

Breakfast _____ Lunch _____ Dinner _____ Snack _____

Meal _____

_____

_____ Glucose _____

---

MY PNP™ MEAL DISCOVERY CARD

Date _____ Pancreas Friendly_____ NOT_____

Breakfast _____ Lunch _____ Dinner _____ Snack _____

Meal _____

_____

_____ Glucose _____

---

MY PNP™ MEAL DISCOVERY CARD

Date _____ Pancreas Friendly_____ NOT_____

Breakfast _____ Lunch _____ Dinner _____ Snack _____

Meal _____

_____

_____ Glucose _____

MY PNP™ MEAL DISCOVERY CARD

Date _____ Pancreas Friendly_____ NOT_____

Breakfast _____ Lunch _____ Dinner _____ Snack _____

Meal _____

_____

_____ Glucose _____

MY PNP™ MEAL DISCOVERY CARD

Date _____ Pancreas Friendly_____ NOT_____

Breakfast _____ Lunch _____ Dinner _____ Snack _____

Meal _____

_____

_____ Glucose _____

MY PNP™ MEAL DISCOVERY CARD

Date _____ Pancreas Friendly_____ NOT_____

Breakfast _____ Lunch _____ Dinner _____ Snack _____

Meal _____

_____

_____ Glucose _____

## MY PNP™ MEAL DISCOVERY CARD

Date _____ Pancreas Friendly____ NOT____

Breakfast ____ Lunch ____ Dinner ____ Snack ____

Meal _____

_____

_____ Glucose _____

## MY PNP™ MEAL DISCOVERY CARD

Date _____ Pancreas Friendly____ NOT____

Breakfast ____ Lunch ____ Dinner ____ Snack ____

Meal _____

_____

_____ Glucose _____

## MY PNP™ MEAL DISCOVERY CARD

Date _____ Pancreas Friendly____ NOT____

Breakfast ____ Lunch ____ Dinner ____ Snack ____

Meal _____

_____

_____ Glucose _____

MY PNP™ MEAL DISCOVERY CARD

Date _____ Pancreas Friendly_____ NOT_____

Breakfast _____ Lunch _____ Dinner _____ Snack _____

Meal _____

_____

_____ Glucose _____

MY PNP™ MEAL DISCOVERY CARD

Date _____ Pancreas Friendly_____ NOT_____

Breakfast _____ Lunch _____ Dinner _____ Snack _____

Meal _____

_____

_____ Glucose _____

MY PNP™ MEAL DISCOVERY CARD

Date _____ Pancreas Friendly_____ NOT_____

Breakfast _____ Lunch _____ Dinner _____ Snack _____

Meal _____

_____

_____ Glucose _____

MY PNP™ MEAL DISCOVERY CARD

Date _____ Pancreas Friendly_____ NOT_____

Breakfast _____ Lunch _____ Dinner _____ Snack _____

Meal _____

_____

_____ Glucose _____

MY PNP™ MEAL DISCOVERY CARD

Date _____ Pancreas Friendly_____ NOT_____

Breakfast _____ Lunch _____ Dinner _____ Snack _____

Meal _____

_____

_____ Glucose _____

MY PNP™ MEAL DISCOVERY CARD

Date _____ Pancreas Friendly_____ NOT_____

Breakfast _____ Lunch _____ Dinner _____ Snack _____

Meal _____

_____

_____ Glucose _____

MY PNP™ MEAL DISCOVERY CARD

Date _____ Pancreas Friendly____ NOT____

Breakfast ____ Lunch ____ Dinner ____ Snack ____

Meal _____

_____

_____ Glucose _____

---

MY PNP™ MEAL DISCOVERY CARD

Date _____ Pancreas Friendly____ NOT____

Breakfast ____ Lunch ____ Dinner ____ Snack ____

Meal _____

_____

_____ Glucose _____

---

MY PNP™ MEAL DISCOVERY CARD

Date _____ Pancreas Friendly____ NOT____

Breakfast ____ Lunch ____ Dinner ____ Snack ____

Meal _____

_____

_____ Glucose _____

MY PNP™ MEAL DISCOVERY CARD

Date _____ Pancreas Friendly____ NOT____

Breakfast _____ Lunch _____ Dinner _____ Snack _____

Meal _____

_____

_____ Glucose _____

MY PNP™ MEAL DISCOVERY CARD

Date _____ Pancreas Friendly____ NOT____

Breakfast _____ Lunch _____ Dinner _____ Snack _____

Meal _____

_____

_____ Glucose _____

MY PNP™ MEAL DISCOVERY CARD

Date _____ Pancreas Friendly____ NOT____

Breakfast _____ Lunch _____ Dinner _____ Snack _____

Meal _____

_____

_____ Glucose _____

MY PNP™ MEAL DISCOVERY CARD

Date _____ Pancreas Friendly____ NOT____

Breakfast ____ Lunch ____ Dinner ____ Snack ____

Meal _____

_____

_____ Glucose _____

MY PNP™ MEAL DISCOVERY CARD

Date _____ Pancreas Friendly____ NOT____

Breakfast ____ Lunch ____ Dinner ____ Snack ____

Meal _____

_____

_____ Glucose _____

MY PNP™ MEAL DISCOVERY CARD

Date _____ Pancreas Friendly____ NOT____

Breakfast ____ Lunch ____ Dinner ____ Snack ____

Meal _____

_____

_____ Glucose _____

## MY PNP™ MEAL DISCOVERY CARD

Date _____ Pancreas Friendly____ NOT____

Breakfast ____ Lunch ____ Dinner ____ Snack ____

Meal _____

_____

_____ Glucose _____

---

## MY PNP™ MEAL DISCOVERY CARD

Date _____ Pancreas Friendly____ NOT____

Breakfast ____ Lunch ____ Dinner ____ Snack ____

Meal _____

_____

_____ Glucose _____

---

## MY PNP™ MEAL DISCOVERY CARD

Date _____ Pancreas Friendly____ NOT____

Breakfast ____ Lunch ____ Dinner ____ Snack ____

Meal _____

_____

_____ Glucose _____

# About the Author

**Candice Rosen, R.N., B.S., M.S.W., C.H.C.**
**Founder, Executive Director and Principal PNP™**
**Health Counselor**

As a Registered Nurse with a Master's Degree in Social Work and Certification in Health Counseling from the Institute for Integrative Nutrition, Candice Rosen has spent her life's work focused on improving the wellness of both her clients and her community. Her experiences as a clinical therapist and as a nurse give her a unique perspective when it comes to nutrition counseling. Candice has an innate understanding of the medical and psychological components that must be addressed in order to achieve health goals and targeted weight loss results.

As the founding member of Gilda's Club Chicago and its first executive director and program director, Candice created and coordinated a diverse array of wellness-related programming. Now Chair of Healthcare Initiatives for Chicago's Sister Cities International Program, she works to advocate preventive medicine, increase maternal and infant health care, improve disability access, promote nourishing diets, and bring awareness to the obesity and diabetes epidemics that now affects populations on a global level.

The originator and director of the Pancreatic Nutritional Program™ (PNP™), Candice is also on a mission to educate the general public as to the crucial role the pancreas plays in overall health, wellness and maintaining an optimal weight. She was inspired to write this, her second book, *The Pancreatic Oath* (Spring 2011), based on her experience helping many clients with conditions such as diabetes, cardiovascular disease, obesity, metabolic syndrome, polycystic ovarian syndrome, and kidney disease. She has helped to manage and often reverse their symptoms through her innovative Pancreatic Nutritional Program™. Too often the accepted method of practice is to treat symptoms with prescription drugs, while ignoring underlying causes. The PNP™ and this book focus on the underlying causes, specifically pancreatic abuse, and treat the source of illness rather than the consequences. While Candice stresses that there is no such thing as a "one size fits all" diet, she has developed a program that benefits all who practice it.

## EDUCATION

Institute For Integrative Nutrition and the State
University of New York (SUNY), New York City,
New York—Certified Health Coach

Loyola University, Chicago, Illinois—Master of Social
Work

University of St. Francis, Joliet, Illinois—Bachelor of
Science

South Chicago Community Hospital School of Nursing,
Chicago, Illinois—Registered Nurse

## LICENSURE

Licensed Social Worker—State of Illinois

Licensed Registered Nurse—State of Illinois

## PROFESSIONAL AND COMMUNITY INVOLVEMENT

Chairman, Healthcare Initiatives, Chicago Sister Cities
International Program

Board of Directors, Chicago Sister Cities International
Program

Member, Access Living's Major Gifts Campaign
Committee

Member, Ambassador Council, Center for Integrative
Medicine and Wellness, Northwestern University
Medical Center

Board Member, Face the Future Foundation

Member, International Women's Association

Member, American Association of Drugless Practitioners

Member, American Holistic Nurses Association
Member, American Nurses Association
Member, Illinois Nurses Association
Member, National Association of Social Workers
Member, Illinois Society of Clinical Social Work
Member, Illinois Mental Health Association
Member, Association Oncology Social Work
Member, Oncology Nurses Society
Member, Northwestern University Circle Club
Member, Evanston and Glenbrook Hospital Auxiliary
Honoree, Notable Alumni—University of St. Francis 90th
    Anniversary Celebratory Magazine

## FAMILY

Candice and her husband, Steven, have four children, a Portuguese water dog, an African Grey Parrot, and a Red-Eared Slider Turtle.

CPSIA information can be obtained at www.ICGtesting.com
Printed in the USA
LVOW04s1147180914

404701LV00003B/206/P